The Joe Dillon
DIFFERENCE

The Evolution
of Weight Loss

Joe Dillon and Sandy Terrien

ISBN 978-0-9838203-2-1

The Joe Dillon Difference: The Evolution of Weight Loss

The information in this book is presented for educational and informational purposes only. It is not intended to treat disease, serve as medical advice or instruction, or replace the services of healing professionals. It is not intended to diagnose or treat any medical condition or to serve as a substitute for professional medical advice, diagnosis, or treatment. For specific medical advice, diagnosis, or treatment, consult your doctor.

We are not liable for any advice, course of treatment, diagnosis, or any other information, services, or products you may obtain from this publication or from our website. You are encouraged to confer with your doctor with regard to information contained herein and you are encouraged to review the information carefully with your healthcare provider.

Published by Middle River Press
1498 NE 30th Court
Oakland Park, FL 33334
middleriverpress.com

First Printing — Printed in the USA

The Joe Dillon
DIFFERENCE

The Evolution
of Weight Loss

Joe Dillon and Sandy Terrien

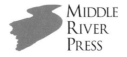
MIDDLE
RIVER
PRESS

To Sandy:
The best lover, friend, and partner I have ever had.
Bun, I couldn't do it without you. Thank you.
—Joe

To Joe:
My love and my partner, without whom
this book would not be possible.
We are so lucky to have found each other!
And to my daughter, Amanda,
the most important woman in my life.
—Sandy (Mom)

Table of Contents

Introduction

Our thesis is that much of the increase in human obesity is due to a mismatch between adaptive biological characteristics and the modern environment.

—Michael L. Power, PhD, and Jay Schulkin, PhD,
The Evolution of Obesity, 2009

Losing weight is a challenge, but the fact that you may struggle with weight is not your fault.

Our goal in writing this book is to help you clearly identify the challenges you face (and they might not be the challenges you expect!), and then show you exactly how to overcome each of them so you can not only lose weight, but also thrive and achieve optimal health.

As the subtitle of this book (The Evolution of Weight Loss) implies, we have a different approach to losing weight. The Joe Dillon Difference lifestyle is a fully integrated weight-loss approach built on a foundation of evolutionary and molecular biology. By anchoring our approach in the biological reality of your body, The Joe Dillon Difference lifestyle is based on the most current scientific research—despite the fact that this may go against conventional wisdom. But rest assured our program is safe, effective and consistent. You'll get the results you intend to produce (effective), and they will be sustainable and predictable (consistent).

With The Joe Dillon Difference lifestyle, you will know exactly what to do and exactly why you are doing it. And don't worry—we will keep it simple and down to earth.

This book is divided into three sections. The first section spells out the major challenges you will meet as you begin your weight-loss program. The second section explains the biological essentials of health for all human beings. In the third section, we will share practical steps you can take to overcome the major challenges to losing weight.

Section One: Major Challenges to Weight Loss

When you begin your weight-loss journey, you'll start off facing a dynamic triad of challenges, including:

- **The interaction of your genes** (your genetic inheritance)
- **Your development**
- **Your environment**

Additional challenges include the aging process, inflammation, and body composition. We'll address each of these in greater depth, but it's especially important to understand body composition. Body composition is a measure of how much of your total body weight is fat and how much is lean body mass (fat-free weight). Optimizing your body composition is the central focus of our program. This is accomplished through managing your insulin levels; maximizing the mobilization of body fat; and burning the maximum amount of body fat.

The Genetic Challenge. Your genetic inheritance is the most deeply rooted challenge you will face on your weight-loss journey. Each of us has our own genetic inheritance. Human beings (*Homo sapiens*) evolved over millions of years to thrive in a very different environment than our modern world. What was advantageous to our early ancestors has become a liability for many of us modern humans today. To express the genetic challenge in simple terms: We evolved in an environment of scarcity and uncertainty—our bodies were programmed to take full advantage of occasional excesses and seasonal times of abundance. Accordingly, our bodies evolved to efficiently store fat as a buffer against times of food shortage and energy deficit.

In the modern environment, however, we find ourselves surrounded by virtually unlimited food. We also evolved in a physically demanding environment that required us to work hard to get the food we needed to stay alive. Not anymore. Today, we live in an environment where we can order pizza while sitting on our couches in front of our TVs. The result of overabundant calories and a lack of physical activity: A global epidemic of excess body fat and its accompanying metabolic diseases, including diabetes and heart disease. This is not merely an American problem. It's common to all industrialized and developing countries. Rapidly developing countries such as India and China are experiencing similar epidemics of diabetes and obesity.

All humans were dealt this same genetic challenge "deck of cards"—it's not unique to any geography or family or ethnicity. Not understanding this genetic challenge leads to futile and self-defeating attempts at weight loss. About 98 percent of all people who go on diets end up fatter than ever. But that doesn't mean it's hopeless. If you learn to play your cards more skillfully, you can compensate for your genetic inheritance and lose weight while thriving and achieving optimal health.

The Developmental Challenge. The second component of the gene/development/environment triad is the developmental challenge. Each of us was conceived and grew in our mother's womb. Early development (starting with conception and continuing past weaning) is also a major challenge to weight loss. What do we mean? Just as each of us has our genetic inheritance, we each have our epigenetic inheritance. Epigenetic changes are not changes in our genes. Epigenetic changes are changes in the *expression* of our genes. In simple terms, your epigenome is responsible for turning genes "on" and "off," like a series of switches.

Epigenetic changes come about when our genes interact with our environment. Major scientific research beginning in the 1980s has shown that adaptations made during conception, embryonic, fetal, neonatal, and childhood development have lifelong consequences in terms of body fat accumulation and the long-term risk of metabolic diseases such as diabetes, hypertension and heart disease (Barker et al 1998; West-Eberhard 2003; Barker 2008). During certain critical windows, epigenetic "decisions" are made with permanent, long-term consequences.

How can this be? Fundamentally, during our early development (starting in the womb), our growing body fine-tunes our gene expression in an

attempt to better match our biology to the environment our bodies anticipate being born into. This is called *developmental plasticity* (West-Eberhard
2003). There are certain critical windows during which the developing em-
bryo/fetus/child makes irreversible biological decisions about its physiology and life-growth trajectory.

Starting literally at conception, the developing child reads cues from
the maternal environment and tries to predict what sort of a world it will
be born into. Based upon these cues, the developing child makes irreversible predictions and changes its physiology accordingly. If the developing
child guesses right, the predictive adaptive responses are advantageous and
the emerging child thrives (Gluckman and Hanson 2005; Gluckman and
Hanson, 2008; Gluckman et al. 2009). But if the developing child misreads
the cues or is given inaccurate cues by the maternal environment, then the
child guesses wrong and the irreversible physiologic changes it makes end
up being inappropriate to its environment. The result is a metabolic mismatch (Gluckman and Hanson 2008), and the child is mismatched with
its postnatal environment. For example, if a developing child is undernourished during pregnancy, the developing child will predict that it will be
born into a nutritionally deprived environment. The result is a low birth
weight baby. This low birth weight baby is metabolically mismatched with
our modern environment of abundance and excess. The consequences of
this metabolic mismatch will grow worse as the child grows and advances
into middle and old age. Some consequences of this metabolic mismatch
include childhood and adult obesity, insulin resistance, diabetes, and heart
disease (Barker 1998).

The moral of this story? The time to begin giving a child the best possible chance to thrive in life is literally before conception. Failure to take
advantage of this critical developmental window is an opportunity that is
lost forever. Obesity, diabetes, and other metabolic diseases are set in mo-
tion before a child is even born (Gluckman et al. 2010).

The Environmental Challenge. The third component of the gene/develop-
ment/environment triad is environmental. We can't change our genetics,
and we can't change how we developed in our mother's womb or our early
childhood. But we can learn how to change and control our environment.
We can learn how to modify our behavior to manage the genetic and developmental cards we were dealt.

The environment we were born into impacts us in a multitude of ways. We first learn how, what, when, and how much to eat from the people who raise us. Many of us learn about nutrition in our school environment: in class, from our peers, and from the food choices available to us at school. We also learn from commercials on television (one of the most powerful advertising tools ever invented). Commercials tell us how to eat, what to eat, when to eat, and why to eat certain foods—and the reasons we are given are seldom related to health.

Television marketing exploits *cephalic responses*. Cephalic responses are the ways our brain responds to the sight, smell, thought, and taste of food and, in turn, how our brain prepares our body to eat. A classic example of a cephalic response can be found in Pavlov's famous dog. As you may recall, Dr. Pavlov conditioned his dog by ringing a bell and then feeding the dog. He did this over and over again. Over time, the dog so strongly associated the sound of the bell ringing with food that all Dr. Pavlov had to do was ring the bell and his dog started salivating in anticipation of food. The dog's salivation was not caused by food or eating. There was no food present. The dog's salivation was caused 100 percent by its brain's response to the anticipation of food.

There are powerful brain-gut links between the sight, smell, taste, or even anticipation of food and our motivation to eat. This is what gives TV ads their mouthwatering power—they are not working on your true need for healthy food, but on your conditioned response to programmed food-related stimuli. Like Pavlov's dog, we have been trained to crave a diet that is high-calorie, high-fat, high-sugar, and yet deficient in many essential macro and micronutrients. As a result, many of us are overfed but undernourished.

The environmental challenge is compounded by the fact that our modern environment requires little or no physical effort to attain food. Here's the reality: We live in an *obesogenic environment*. An obesogenic environment is an environment that literally encourages obesity and its associated metabolic disorders (e.g., inflammation, diabetes, and heart disease).

Unfortunately, the fault for this doesn't just lie with fast-food restaurants and junk food manufacturers, which reap huge profits from the current system. And besides, you can't expect junk food manufacturers or fast-food restaurants to change. The problem is that even the official U.S. government–approved Food Pyramid/The Plate, which is guaranteed to make you fat, tired, and depressed with its heavy emphasis on carbohydrates, is complicit. So as a result, many of us eat more carbohydrates than we can handle metabolically (Reaven 2001).

The result of this triad is a devastating epidemic of obesity and the diseases associated with obesity. In the United States, the Centers for Disease Control estimates that about 67 percent of all adult Americans are overweight. Ninety million Americans are obese.

As just one person, you can't change the entrenched interests that work against us. The only thing you can change is you. You have control over your environment and your behavior. We are here to help you make constructive and effective changes to produce the weight loss you want.

The Aging Challenge. Why does it get harder to lose weight as we age? There are lots of reasons. To name just a few, we lose lean body mass (muscle), which burns fat and calories; our metabolism slows down; and we become more glucose intolerant (carbohydrate intolerant) and more insulin resistant. Aging, therefore, is a major challenge to losing weight. Unfortunately, no one can stop the aging process. But it has been well established that we can either speed up the aging process with unwise lifestyle habits, or we can significantly slow down the aging process with proactive lifestyle habits (Rosenburg and Evans 1990).

The Inflammation Challenge. Inflammation is a silent challenge caused by the metabolic mismatch of our genetic inheritance, our developmental inheritance, our modern obesogenic environment and diet, stress, and excess body fat. If you don't know what you are looking for (inflammation) or how to go about looking for inflammation, you might not realize you are struggling with the major challenge of inflammation. In 2004, *Time* magazine called inflammation the "silent killer." Fortunately, there are precise scientific methods to measure the level of inflammatory molecules in your body.

Inflammation, just like everything else in your body, is molecular. The most conclusive and inarguable proof of elevated inflammation levels is a full inflammation marker panel, which is taken as part of a comprehensive set of blood tests. These blood tests precisely measure the levels of all four major inflammation markers and compares these levels to the optimal ranges.

The symptoms of chronic inflammation include everything from acid reflux and asthma to degenerative diseases such as heart disease. Some of us have a greater genetic or developmental tendency to inflammation. Fortunately, inflammation can be virtually 100 percent controlled by a healthy lifestyle. Our clients following The Joe Dillon Difference lifestyle have achieved optimal inflammation markers in just ninety days. Without drugs.

What does inflammation have to do with weight loss? As you will learn, adipose tissue (fat tissue) functions as an endocrine organ. Our body fat secretes literally dozens of different molecules affecting our body. Some of these molecules are inflammatory cytokines. Inflammatory cytokines cause inflammation on a molecular level. So you see how the connection works: The higher a person's body fat, the more adipose tissue they have. The more adipose tissue a person has, the bigger this endocrine organ and, therefore, the more inflammatory cytokines their body produces. Controlling inflammation is just one of many reasons why leaner is better.

The Body Composition Challenge. Not all weight loss is equal—the true challenge is to optimize your *body composition*. In plain language, your challenge is to lose the right *kind* of weight.

Losing weight indiscriminately will NOT give you the benefits you want. Losing weight indiscriminately will only result in a smaller version of your former self. If you want to look better, be more attractive, feel better, have more energy, and achieve optimal health, you must optimize your body composition. You do this by losing body fat and simultaneously enhancing your lean body mass. The result: You get leaner.

The leaner you get, the better you look.

The leaner you get, the more attractive you are.

The leaner you get, the more energy you have.

The leaner you get, the better you feel.

The leaner you get, the healthier you are.

We will teach you exactly how to lose body fat while simultaneously enhancing your lean body mass.

Section Two: Biological Essentials

Health is molecular.

What does this mean? In order to live and thrive, all living organisms, including human beings, need certain essential molecules. The need for these molecules is non-negotiable. Related to the need for specific molecules is the fact that we age from the brain down. One characteristic that distinguishes human beings from all other species on earth is our big brain. The human brain is an amazing organ, but it's also high maintenance (Aiello and Wheeler 1995).

Biological Essential: Oxygen. The most essential of all molecules necessary for human life is oxygen. It took literally billions of years for our oxygen-rich atmosphere to form. Without an oxygen-rich atmosphere, humans would not exist. Deprive our brains of oxygen for more than four or five minutes, and we die. That is how essential the molecule oxygen is to human health. Quite simply, our challenge is to ensure that a generous amount of oxygen is supplied to our brain and our body at all times. By the same token, we want to avoid anything that might interfere with the process of supplying every single one of the 100 trillion cells in our body with oxygen. And finally, an abundance of oxygen is absolutely crucial to the fat-burning process and, therefore, to the optimization of your body composition.

Oxygen is essential to getting lean.

Biological Essential: Water. H_2O is the second most essential molecule. It took 500 million years for the hydrosphere to form on earth. That is, it took 500 million years after the formation of the earth 4.6 billion years ago for the planet to become the watery planet we know today (70 percent of the earth's surface is covered with water). Without water, there would be no life. Even in a temperate climate, human beings can only go for about four or five days without pure water or we die. Of all our organs, our brain is the most devastated by dehydration. After getting enough oxygen, drinking optimal amounts of pure water is the second most important element in losing weight and achieving optimal health. If that's not enough incentive, the number one cause of memory loss at any age is dehydration.

Biological Essential: Lean Protein. Protein is the next most important set of essential molecules for optimal health and weight loss. The earliest precursors to all life on our planet were organic protein molecules. Our genes (DNA via RNA) encode proteins.

Protein is so important that these molecules are called the eight "essential" amino acids. The eight essential amino acids are the fundamental building blocks from which our body makes literally thousands of other proteins. For genes to synthesize proteins, they need these essential building blocks. Proteins, in turn, are the workhorses of our human body. From muscles to bones to enzymes to hormones, proteins carry out our life processes.

It is important to eat the highest quality sources of these eight essential amino acids, which means eating lean, complete proteins multiple times a day. Lean, complete protein containing all eight essential amino acids is so important to human development that pregnant women, lactating women, and growing children need 50 percent more lean, complete protein than the rest of us.

We will teach you exactly how to eat to ensure that you and your family obtain optimal amounts of lean, complete protein.

Biological Essential: Essential Fat. Omega-3 fat is essential to human health. The cell membrane of every single cell in your body is made out of fat (phospholipids).

Not just any fat, essential fat. There are two essential fats: omega-3 and omega-6. In ideal circumstances, they are represented in your diet in a specific ratio. Unfortunately, most people's diets are way out of balance, with too much omega-6 and virtually no omega-3.

Omega-3 fat is also crucial for the development and health of the 100 billion cells in your brain. Omega-3 fat is so important for brain development that pregnant women, lactating women, and growing children need 50 percent more omega-3 fat than the rest of us. We will teach you how to eat and supplement to ensure that you and your family get optimal amounts of essential omega-3 fat.

Biological Essential: Low Glycemic Load Carbohydrates. Our human brain is one of the most high-maintenance organs in the universe. In most cases, our brain can only burn the molecule glucose for fuel. In fact, your brain burns over 20 percent of the glucose consumed by your body every twenty-four hours. This is one reason we all have a sweet tooth.

But your brain is also very fussy. It's a bit like Goldilocks: It doesn't want too much glucose; it doesn't want too little glucose; it wants your glucose level to be just right. Unfortunately, because of this sweet tooth and the easy availability of processed carbohydrates, most of us eat far too many carbohydrates—and most of these are processed carbohydrates, the worst kind. You love carbohydrates, but they don't love you.

The optimal sources of glucose are *low glycemic load carbohydrates* combined with lean, complete proteins (Liu et al. 2002). Low glycemic load carbohydrates break down the slowest and raise your insulin the least. Insulin is the hormone that moves glucose from your bloodstream into your cells. The more carbohydrates you eat, the higher your insulin levels are as your body works to clear glucose from the bloodstream (carbohydrates are converted into glucose in your body).

Insulin management is a key component to losing weight and optimizing your body composition. We will teach you the kinds of foods to eat in what combinations to ensure your blood sugar is stable twenty-four hours a day (and that your insulin levels are optimal). Stable blood sugar levels and low levels of insulin are crucial to burning fat and optimal health. Any time you spike your insulin, fat burning grinds to a halt for the next 8 to 12 hours – even if you exercise. Combine optimal amounts of lean, complete protein to build muscle and bone with moderate amounts of low glycemic load carbohydrates, and you will get leaner and healthier with no hunger and no cravings.

Biological Essential: Full Body Aerobic Exercise. Another biological essential is activity, or exercise. The most important kind of exercise is aerobic exercise. Aerobic means "with air" or "with oxygen." The more oxygen you get to the cells of your body, the more fat you burn. The more oxygen you get to the cells of your body, the more energy you will have.

The most effective kind of aerobic exercise is full-body aerobic exercise. The more lean body mass you involve in your aerobic exercise, the more you stimulate your metabolism. Full-body aerobic exercise strengthens and enhances your cardiovascular system, including your heart, your lungs, and your circulatory system.

Bottom line: To burn more fat and have more energy, you need a big, strong, athletic heart. Your body does not lie. A very simple measure of the strength of your heart is your resting heart rate. The amount of energy you have is a function of the strength and fitness of your cardiovascular system. We will teach you a simple, practical, and effective full-body aerobic exercise you can do in your home, around your neighborhood, or on a treadmill at your gym. The exercise we will teach you will get you into your best aerobic shape in years—perhaps ever. It will also accelerate your metabolism, so you will burn more fat and more calories twenty-four hours a day, and it will also reduce insulin resistance.

Biological Essential: Optimal Sleep. Recovery is just as important as exercise. Sleep is an integral component of the recovery process. Optimal sleep is crucial to burning fat and building muscle. In fact, optimal sleep is so important that lack of sleep (chronic exhaustion) actually makes people fatter. We will teach you exactly how to get a sound night's sleep—regardless of your age. For the record, it is a myth we need less sleep as we get older. We always need an optimal amount of sleep, but as we get older, it just gets harder to achieve.

It may surprise you to learn we recommend eating your very last meal 30–60 minutes before you turn off your light and go to sleep. Never go to bed hungry. Why? If your blood sugar is stable, you will sleep longer and more soundly. But it is important to avoid over-carbing at dinner and at your pre-sleep meal. If you avoid carbs before bed, you will also burn more fat and build more muscle while you sleep.

Biological Essential: Supplementation. We encourage you to eat real, whole, unprocessed foods in small to moderate size meals, four to six times a day. But even eating an optimal diet, you will still not be able to attain optimal amounts of *all* the nutrients your body needs to thrive. To fill this gap, we will encourage you to take a few pharmaceutical-grade supplements.

To be clear, supplements are NOT substitutes. There is no supplement on earth that can replace oxygen, water, the eight essential amino acids, full-body aerobic exercise, or optimal sleep. But pure, pharmaceutical-grade supplements can give you that last 5 percent.

Section Three: Effective Actions

The final section of the book deals with effective actions you can take as part of The Joe Dillon Difference lifestyle. Once you've learned the underlying reasons—how to confront your challenges, how your body optimally operates—we will then provide you with concrete steps to put it all into action.

Effective Action: Set YOUR Personal Goals. An essential step in losing weight is to clearly define your destination. As the saying goes, "If you don't know where you are going, any road will do."

Clearly defining your destination means setting a positive, measurable goal with a deadline. Since your primary goal is weight loss, your single most important task is to determine your true ideal body weight. There is only one accurate scientific method to determine your true ideal body weight—and it's not using your body mass index (BMI).

First, you must determine your body composition, or your ratio of body fat to lean body mass. The ideal body fat percentage for men is 15 percent or less and 22 percent or less for women. Once you know this, you can calculate your true ideal body weight by adding your optimal amount of body fat to your optimal lean body mass (your fat-free weight). This is unique to YOUR body.

You can then calculate how long it will take you to lose your excess body fat until you reach your ideal weight. We will help you accurately manage your expectations.

Effective Action: Control YOUR Environment. To lose weight, it is crucial to create a controlled environment (or environments) conducive to weight loss. Remember, environment is a component of the dynamic triad (genes/development/environment) of challenges. A simple but powerful fact of the reality of weight loss is this: If it is in your house, you (and your family) will eat it.

We will give you crystal clear directions as to what to eliminate from your home, and more importantly, we will give you four lists of what to include: pure water; lean, complete proteins; healthy fats; and low glycemic load (slow-burning) carbohydrates.

Effective Action: Control YOUR Day. This is YOUR day. Take charge of YOUR day. You will NEVER get this day again. We will give you a template for an optimally healthy day, so you can take full advantage of YOUR day. We will spell out a balanced eating plan, including what to eat, when to eat, and how much to eat at each of your small to moderate meals. We will teach you how to integrate exercise into your day, what to eat before you exercise, what to eat after your workout to maximize your benefits from your workout, and how to get a sound night's sleep. Follow these recommendations and you will get leaner; you will create the best blood panel you have ever had; you will have more energy than you have had in years; you will have a sharper mind and memory; and you will look your best. You will be more attractive.

Effective Action: Listen to YOUR Body. The Joe Dillon Difference lifestyle is reality based. We will teach you how to get connected to the reality of your body and how to stay connected. One of the simplest and most direct methods for doing this is to measure your body. We are going to encourage you to take a few simple measurements every day. With a few minutes a day, you will be able to track your progress and fine-tune your process. Each time you measure and write down your results (what gets measured, gets done) you are documenting your progress. We are big believers in black and white, objective evidence that proves and documents your results.

If you follow the plan, you will get leaner, look better, feel better, have more energy, have the best comprehensive blood panel you have ever had in your life, and achieve and sustain optimal health ON PURPOSE. Why? Because you made accurate choices congruent with your biology. And if you continue to make these accurate biological choices, you will continue to enjoy the benefits of vibrant good health for the rest of your long and healthy life.

Effective Action: Manage YOUR Setbacks. We are ALL human (including Sandy and me). That means we all have setbacks and reversals. We all occasionally fall off the wagon. We will teach you how to deal with setbacks and how to bounce back. The Joe Dillon Difference lifestyle is your track to run on. When you get off track, the most important thing is to get right back on track. A fundamental component of thriving is the ability physically, mentally, and emotionally to bounce back.

Conclusion

We all face major challenges when we try to lose weight, starting with the dynamic triad (genes/development/environment). On top of these three major challenges, we are all getting older (sad to say). We are challenged with losing the right kind of weight while trying to enhance our lean body mass. And we face the challenge of inflammation—the silent challenge.

The Joe Dillon Difference will address each of these challenges with recommendations based on sound, uncomplicated science. The Joe Dillon Difference lifestyle is frank and straightforward. Keep it simple. Focus on the basics. Work the problem. Eliminate distractions.

At the end of this book, you will find a list of resources and tools to help you implement and sustain your program. You will also find an extensive bibliography. The Joe Dillon Difference lifestyle is based on peer-reviewed science and empirical data. If you want to pursue any of the issues discussed in this book, we invite you to check out our bibliography. It's a rich source of some of the most up-to-date research available today.

The Bottom Line. This book will teach you how to optimize your body composition (lose the right kind of weight and look your best); how to take first-class care of your brain and avoid many of the cognitive problems associated with aging; how to achieve and sustain optimal health; how to take full advantage of one of human beings' most valuable characteristics: adaptability; how to create a healthy environment for you and your family; and how to age successfully.

Please join us for an interesting and exciting journey.

Our Stories

When the student is ready, the teacher will appear.
—Buddhist proverb

Before we take you on your journey, we want to first share with you our journey and our life story. We hope this will give you some insight into us, and also perhaps some insight into the challenges you may also be experiencing.

We also hope that by sharing our journey with you, you will understand why we are so passionate about what we teach and why we are so confident our program is effective.

Joe Dillon's Story

Let's begin at the beginning. In 1944 (in the midst of the Second World War), I was born in San Francisco, California. My father, a captain in the United States Marine Corps, served in the South Pacific on the island of Okinawa, fighting the Japanese. When World War II ended, he came home. We then moved to the University of California, Davis, where my father finished his college education. He then settled into his career, and we moved to San Mateo, California, a new suburb twenty miles south of San Francisco, where my parents provided our family with a modest, middle class lifestyle, one that might be very similar to yours.

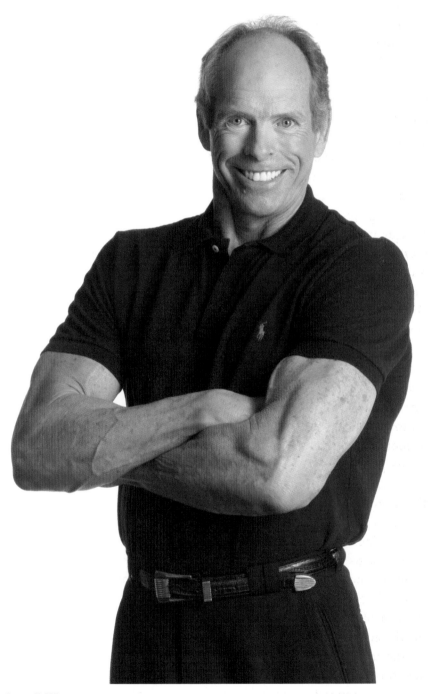

Joe Dillon

When it came to health and lifestyle, unfortunately, my parents were completely trapped in the Black Box of Conventional Wisdom. They bought hook, line, and sinker into what marketing taught us was "the good life." Television, which was just coming of age and which is the most powerful marketing tool ever invented, reinforced this propaganda.

Every night, my family and I dutifully assumed our places at the dining room table, swiveled the television set around, and watched our favorite programs while we ate. We became devoted disciples of television marketing. Like automatons, we went out and bought everything TV ads told us was required if we were to enjoy "the good life." Each morning, we began our daily rituals of "the good life" by drinking a big glass of reconstituted, frozen orange juice. We filled big bowls with "whole grain" cereal coated with sugar and poured the "perfect" food, whole milk, over our frosted cereal. Or we drank cups of hot chocolate made from a can of powder mixed into whole milk with some whipped cream out of a can and ate boxes of white powdered-sugar donuts.

On the weekends, we had time for a more elaborate breakfast. My father did the honors. First, he fried a pound of bacon while he smoked cigarettes and drank coffee. Then he fried eggs in the bacon grease and ladled the bacon grease over the eggs. He called them "basted eggs." He saved the leftover bacon grease in a coffee can. My mother used the bacon grease to fry the rest of our meals. Along with bacon and basted eggs, we ate white bread toast slathered with butter and jam or jelly. Breakfast over, my parents smoked cigarettes and drank coffee. My dad read the sports section. Both my parents smoked two packs of cigarettes a day. They did no real exercise except for occasionally working in the garden on the weekends. In addition, my father played golf once a month.

My mother prepared the rest of the meals. She had grown up in a family of nine children. Her father was a police officer in San Francisco. He was shot to death by a robber when my mother was nine years old. Her mother, now a widow, raised all nine children by herself on a ranch in Napa Valley during the Great Depression. They did not have much. As a result of her upbringing, my mother prepared solid meals in huge quantities and served them family style: big bowls and platters in the center of the table. Typical dinners included: hot dogs, canned beans, and canned brown bread with lots of butter; tuna noodle casserole made with canned tuna; canned Spam baked with canned pineapple slices; frozen fish sticks and applesauce from a jar; big greasy cheeseburgers made with cheap hamburger on white bread buns with sliced tomatoes and iceberg lettuce dripping with mayonnaise and ketchup; chicken deep-fat fried in bacon grease with homemade biscuits and gravy. We had the same salad with every dinner: iceberg lettuce, sliced tomatoes, and radishes. We had the same dressing on every salad: Thousand Island dressing made with mayonnaise and ketchup. At every meal, my mother prepared more than enough food. Everyone could eat as much as they wanted to eat. We all had seconds and even thirds.

We ended every meal with my mother's homemade desserts: chocolate chip cookies, chocolate cake, apple pie, peach cobbler, or brownies with chocolate frosting. We ate every dessert with ice cream—generous slabs of vanilla or chocolate. There was always enough dessert for seconds and thirds. As my mother so often said: "A meal without dessert is not a balanced meal." How did we know when a meal was over? When we couldn't take another bite.

Sunday evening we had our special meal for the week: pot roast, mashed potatoes and gravy; or leg of lamb with mint jelly, plus baked potatoes drowned in butter and sour cream.

Two dynamics were present at every meal: one explicit and one implicit. The explicit dynamic: My parents wanted me to grow up big and strong. As a result, my father served the food and I had to clean my plate at every meal. When I was young, this was a battle. I simply could not eat all the food he gave me. But as I grew older, I had no trouble cleaning my plate and asking for seconds and even thirds. I am still a "clean plate" eater to this day. After all, as my mother was so fond of saying: "There are people starving in China."

The implicit dynamic was love. Because my mother loved me, she fixed big, hearty meals. My end of the bargain was simple: If I loved my mother, I would demonstrate my love by eating generous amounts of the food she had prepared. The more I loved my mother, the more of her food I would eat. My father also participated in this implicit dynamic. And it was not a chore. My mother's food, though not fancy, was solid and good tasting. We all became competitive eaters. As I grew older and bigger, we ate faster and faster, so we could get even more of the food in the big bowls and on the big platters in the center of the table.

The result? We all got fat. Over time, my mother, who was five feet, seven inches tall and who had been a lean, active tomboy when she grew up on the ranch in Napa, grew to over two hundred pounds. My father, who was five feet, nine inches tall and who had been a varsity athlete and then a fitness instructor in the United States Marine Crops, grew to over 250 pounds. I grew fat along with my parents.

Until I was sixteen years old, I was a fat non-athlete. I was one of those fat, clumsy kids always chosen last when kids pick sides. In addition, I was eating so much sugar that I suffered from attention deficit and blood sugar crashes. Few people knew what ADD (attention deficit disorder, or as it is known today, ADHD) was back in the 1950s. So even though I am pretty smart, I got lousy grades and got into a lot of trouble. I spent a lot of time in the principal's office. After school, I hung out with other dysfunctional, ADD kids. We got arrested for shoplifting and vandalism.

No one seemed to understand it or talk about it at the time, but I knew something was wrong. While attending grammar school, I used to grab my big glass of orange juice and chug it down. Then I would eat four or five powdered sugar donuts and wash them down with hot chocolate and jump on my bike and ride to school. Before the first hour of class was over, I would break out in a cold sweat, and I found it nearly impossible to pay attention. I felt weak, shaky, and light-headed. I did not understand until decades later how glucose intolerant I was. I did not understand how much my genetic inheritance and my development played havoc with my metabolism. And I really didn't get how eating massive amounts of sugar and refined carbohydrates exacerbated my metabolic mismatch. I was poorly mismatched with our modern environment and "the good life."

One of my favorite expressions is the Buddhist proverb, "When the student is ready, the teacher will appear." I swam my first two years of high school, but the most you could say was that I made the team. But at the start of my junior year, we got a new coach. He was to be the football coach in the fall and the swimming coach in the spring. The new coach's name? Dick Vermeil. Any football fan knows Dick Vermeil is one of the greatest football coaches of all time. For those of you unfamiliar with football, Coach Vermeil coached UCLA to a huge upset victory in the 1975 Rose Bowl Game against a heavily favored, undefeated, and number one ranked Ohio State team. Coach Vermeil then coached the Philadelphia Eagles to Super Bowl XV. He was named NFL Coach of the Year that year. Later, he coached the St. Louis Rams to victory in Super Bowl

XXXIV. For the second time, Coach Vermeil was voted the best coach in all of professional football. With Dick Vermeil's coaching, I became a high school All-American swimmer. To say Coach Vermeil transformed my life is an understatement.

Upon graduation from high school, I went to junior college, where I was an All-American swimmer as well. At the end of my sophomore year in college, my father died of a massive heart attack. He was 46 years old. My father was a classic example of an unfortunate fact: In 45 percent of cases, the first symptom of heart disease is sudden death. My father's death blind-sided me. I had breakfast with my dad that morning. My final living image of my dad is this: He's sitting at the kitchen table, chain-smoking cigarettes, drinking coffee, and engrossed in the sports page. That was the last time I saw him alive.

After my dad's death, I dropped out of school and joined the United States Marine Corps. That was 1965. The Vietnam War was just beginning to escalate. Like the Second World War was to my father, I felt like Vietnam was my generation's war. I went through boot camp at MCRD (Marine Corps Recruit Depot) San Diego and infantry training at Camp Pendleton, California. Having qualified as an expert swimmer, I got orders to be a fitness instructor in Staging Battalion at Main Side, Camp Pendleton. I taught fitness and survival classes and what was called "combat swim." Despite being a former All-American swimmer, I completed the most challenging and intensive training course I have ever been through in my life: drown proofing. Upon graduation, I was certified as one of the first drown proofing instructors in the United States Marine Corps. Drown proofing is a simple and effective swimming technique. When a ship sinks or a plane goes down out at sea, drown proofing enables a serviceman to survive with no boat, life raft, or floatation device of any kind for days on end. I taught people how to save their lives.

In the fall of 1966, I got my orders, and by September, I was on my way to Vietnam on the aircraft carrier *LPH Valley Forge* as part of what the Marine Corps called vertical envelopment. Very simply, a company or battalion of marines would be heli-lifted off one of these special aircraft carriers and inserted wherever they were needed in a combat zone. Over two thousand of us marines, all specially trained to be inserted into hot spots in the Vietnam combat zone, were on board. We stopped along the way for intense training, first in the Hawaiian Islands, then in Okinawa, and then on to the Philippine Islands. Each day, we faced grueling marches with full combat gear, set up ambushes and killing zones, and learned how to move through the jungle and hunt in packs. We got filthy dirty and exhausted. We grew tougher and meaner. Brutal and demanding as this training was, it turned out to be mild compared to what was to come. Whenever we got liberty, which was not often, we got drunk and let off some of the growing tension building in marines on their way to war.

We landed at Da Nang, the huge marine air base in South Vietnam. I will never forget my first night at Da Nang. I began to grasp that war is a dirty, nasty, twenty-four-hour-a-day, seven-days-a-week job with no weekends off and none of the glory depicted in the John Wayne movies I had been raised on. The flurry of activity at Da Nang air base was massive, overwhelming, and deafening. F-4 Phantom jets roared down the runways day and night on bombing runs and providing close air support for the grunts (marines fighting on the ground). The jet engines were so loud it was literally visceral. At night, the flames shooting out of the back of the jets looked both terrible and spectacular. Heavy artillery pounded out fire missions. I hardly slept a wink.

We got orders to Dong Ha. I had heard of Da Nang, but I had never heard of Dong Ha. Dong Ha, as it turned out, was the southeast corner of what became known as Leatherneck Square where some of the most intense fighting took place in Vietnam. Dong Ha was only a few miles south of the misnamed Demilitarized Zone (DMZ). The North Vietnamese shelled and rocketed Dong Ha on a regular basis. Dong Ha turned out to be significantly more dangerous than Da Nang. And, ironically, Dong Ha was to be our "rear," meaning Dong Ha was the safest place we would get to go back to over the next year. And we only got back to Dong Ha a couple of times in the next twelve months for a much-needed shower and to replace our filthy, tattered jungle fatigues. The rest of my tour, we fought deep in the jungle and lived in the hole we dug each night. No tent. No sleeping bag. A poncho was all you got.

We wanted action. Be careful what you ask for. We got all the action we could handle. Once in-country, the intensity of combat steadily escalated. Every day, we were attacked with a variety of methods: mortar attacks, rocket attacks, heavy artillery barrages, human wave attacks, and sappers with satchel charges strapped to their bodies to blow a hole in our defensive perimeter. I had never experienced such complete and utter terror in my life. We stood two-man watches: two hours on and two hours off. You were lucky if you got four hours sleep a night. Utterly exhausted, my cigarette habit quickly grew from a pack a day to three or four packs a day. I lit my next cigarette with the butt of the last one. Soon, all the fingers of both of my hands were yellow with nicotine. We went weeks and weeks without a shower or a change of clothes. Our bodies so reeked with the smell of stale sweat and filth that even the clouds of voracious mosquitoes began to leave us alone. Our once-green camouflage trousers literally turned brown with ground-in dirt and grease. With no soap and water, every nick and cut got infected.

Within my first six weeks in-country, over half of my company of two hundred marines had been killed or wounded. I was shot twice during my tour in Vietnam. I had just two weeks left on my tour when I got shot the second time. We were at Con Thien, the northernmost outpost in South Vietnam. Con Thien over looked the so-called DMZ. In reality, the DMZ was a staging area for the North Vietnamese Army. Our mission was to find a break in the North Vietnamese trench line. I was shot through my right thigh by an AK-47 at one o'clock in the afternoon. One after another, my men were blown up and killed. I laid there unable to walk, a tourniquet around my thigh, convinced I would never get out alive. I will never forget the moment when the medevac helicopter cleared the land and flew out over the South China Sea. For the first time in over a year, I knew I was going to get out of Vietnam alive. I have never felt so thankful or so relieved in my entire life.

After spending about ten days on the hospital ship *Repose*, and another couple of weeks at the U.S. Air Force hospital in the Philippines, I was flown to Travis Air Force Base near San Francisco, California. The reality that I had actually made it home alive was slowly sinking in. After a year in the jungle, filthy, exhausted, and constantly fighting, being home in the United States seemed like a miracle. I was safe, but I was an ambivalent, emotional mess, torn between guilt and gratitude. I felt guilty because I was alive (survivor guilt) while my buddies were still fighting, getting killed, and wounded in Vietnam, but I was overcome with relief that I had made it out alive. It was going to be a long road back, both mentally and physically.

When I arrived at Long Beach Naval Hospital, the physician examined me and gave me extended basket leave. That meant I was well enough to leave the hospital but too debilitated for active duty. So I was given a cane and sent home to rest until I was healthy enough to return to active duty. Once home, I hobbled around on my cane, which quickly exhausted me. When I was not sleeping on the couch, I spent most of my time at home watching football on TV, chain smoking, and drinking one ice-cold soda after another. I also read a lot: newspapers, magazines, novels, and an occasional nonfiction book.

It was while I was lying on the couch reading a book that I had a major realization: I had always taken my health for granted. Here I was, twenty-three years old and hobbling around on a cane, chain-smoking cigarettes. I stopped smoking cold turkey that very day. That was early 1968. I have never smoked again. I also vowed to get myself back into shape. Once I could walk without the cane, I began to exercise. This was the first time in my life that I had ever exercised entirely on my own. Competitive swimming in high school and junior college, and then the Marine Corps, had provided all of my exercise up to that point in my life. This was a huge turning point. At first, it was all I could do to slowly walk a mile. Then two miles. Then three. Then I gradually began to slowly walk and jog. Progress seemed excruciatingly slow. Eventually, I ran five miles in under thirty-five minutes every day. But I had not changed my eating habits. I was still living on multiple cans of soda a day, mac-n-cheese, bacon and eggs, and fast-food.

I went back to school at the University of California at Irvine in southern California. I was on a mission. I studied hard and graduated with honors. Upon graduation, I went to work for a Fortune 500 company. Again, being highly competitive, I became their number one salesman in the entire United States. But to achieve this level of success, I worked seventy to ninety hours a week, seven days a week. I never took a vacation. Financially, I was doing great. I rewarded myself by going to the best restaurants and eating rich meals, including wine, after-dinner drinks, and heavy desserts. I was living "the good life." But the burnout, workaholic pace I drove myself to keep up began to take its toll.

By the time I was in my early thirties, despite almost daily exercise (I was still running, only slower), I began to get fat. I had nonstop acid indigestion. Now it is called acid reflux. I sucked nonstop on anti-acid tablets. Thirty-six-hour migraine headaches blinded me once or twice a week. I had no energy. I had broken sleep. I woke up in the middle of the night sweaty, fearful, and anxious, and I couldn't get back to sleep for hours. I became chronically exhausted. Then I began to have medical problems. My blood pressure was going through the roof. My total cholesterol was sky high. But what really grabbed my attention were severe chest pains following meals. These pains would literally double me over after a rich meal. This is called angina. My chest pains indicated that I had serious blockage of my coronary arteries. My heart muscle was not getting enough oxygen. I got scared. The fact that my father had dropped dead of a massive heart attack at age forty-six haunted me. Serious physical pain and fear of premature death made me a ready student.

I could not avoid a stark fact: If I did not change my lifestyle, I would never see my fortieth birthday. Motivated by pain and fear, I was on a mission to literally save my life. Right about this time, a guy who had written a terrific book on running dropped dead of a heart attack. It became crystal clear: Exercise alone was not enough. The huge blind spot in my picture of what it meant to be healthy became glaringly obvious: I was clueless about nutrition. Fortunately, one of the most wonderful things I got out of my college education was I had learned how to learn. I began to systematically educate myself on nutrition.

I began to read everything I could get my hands on about nutrition and diet. I was determined to solve the puzzle of truly healthy and life-supporting nutrition. When I first began to seriously research nutrition and what people considered healthy eating, I was confused by conflicting and contradictory information. But as I read more deeply, I got beneath the surface of the latest best-selling, fad diet books. I began to read textbooks written by PhD-level research scientists. Only then did the *essential* pieces of the puzzle of truly healthy nutrition begin to emerge. It became clear to me: Get deep enough (down to the molecular level) and you see a universal, unchanging pattern of human nutrition and optimal health. This pattern of deeply researched human nutrition facts holds true for every single human being on earth.

The first piece of the puzzle of truly optimal health that fell into place was oxygen. It hit me like a bolt of lightning when I realized the obvious: Every single human being on the planet has to breathe oxygen. No exceptions. This insight became the cornerstone of a foundation of non-negotiable scientific facts of biological health. Oxygen is the single most important *essential* molecule for health.

Next came water. Then the eight essential amino acids. As I began to eat in a way that is congruent with our evolved human biochemistry, my body began to thrive. As I emerged from the ignorance and propaganda of the Black Box of Conventional Wisdom promoting the so-called "good life," the change in my health was just short of miraculous. Within ninety days, I lost over thirty pounds—with no hunger and no cravings. All of my indigestion disappeared and has *never* returned. All of my headaches disappeared and have *never* returned. I started sleeping great. My energy came roaring back. I felt like I was a seventeen-year-old All-American swimmer again. Drug-free, I dropped my blood pressure to 110/70. Today, my blood pressure (drug-free) is 90/60. Drug-free, I dropped my sky-high total cholesterol down to an optimal 185 with an HDL of 78. All my chest pains disappeared and have *never* returned. In fact, I got a full body scan at the Cooper Center, and the physicians declared my heart clean as a whistle. Not a trace of heart disease. I felt a lot like I felt in that medevac helicopter that carried me out of Vietnam. I felt like I had dodged a huge bullet. I felt like I had been given yet another chance.

I felt so encouraged, so full of hope, that I could not keep my mouth shut. I told everyone about my health rebirth. I discovered two things: 1) I love sharing what I have learned about exercise, nutrition, and supplementation; and, 2) A lot of people complain of the same health problems I had suffered from. A few people even made positive changes in their lives after hearing my message. I had found my Path. Or as the great teacher Joseph Campbell would say, I had found my Bliss. I was making the world a better place. I was helping people. I was making a positive contribution.

I got so excited about my tangible, empirical results that I quit my job and started my own corporation. That was June 1979. Initially, I did what is technically known as hydrostatic weighing, commonly called the "dunk" test. Scientifically, hydrostatic weighing is the gold standard. It's the most accurate scientific method of measuring body fat percentage. I tested the body fat of five hundred to one thousand clients a month. I did that for years. I have personally tested the body fat of and then explained the results to literally thousands of clients. I then explained how to achieve and sustain their true ideal body weight. I got so good at estimating a person's body fat that if I saw a man in swim trunks or a woman in a two-piece swimsuit, I could accurately estimate their body fat within plus or minus 1 percent.

It was during this period that I began to work intensely with world-class athletes: Twenty-two of my clients have won over sixty Olympic gold medals; some have won Mr. America, Mr. Universe, Mr. Olympia and Ms. Olympia bodybuilding titles; some have won the Ironman World Triathlon Championship in Hawaii; some have won World Power Lifting Championships (one of my clients, at a body weight of 198 pounds, bench-pressed 528 pounds and squatted 775 pounds); some of my clients are in the Pro Football Hall of Fame; some of my clients are Olympic coaches; some of my clients are CEOs of multimillion dollar companies; and some of my clients are self-made billionaires.

As I built a reputation for producing great results, I was invited to speak to athletic teams, corporations, and dental meetings. After several years, I began to focus my energies exclusively on coaching people individually and speaking all over the country. I have shared the message of how to get leaner, perform at a higher level, and be more productive and optimally healthy at literally thousands of seminars. At every seminar, whether to a corporation, a sales team, a group of CEOs or dental professionals, I encourage my audience to ask me any question they want at any time during my talk. If you really want to learn about health, try answering a barrage of questions in front of over five hundred dental professionals, some with masters degrees in biochemistry in addition to their dental degrees. It is a fantastic motivator to stay current with the state-of-the-art scientific research.

However, I have discovered that the most challenging group are people like you and me. By that I mean busy people who are trying to figure out how they can integrate a healthier lifestyle into their busy, demanding schedules. Let me prove to you that it is possible to get leaner and optimally healthy no matter how busy you are. I fly between 100,000 and 200,000 miles a year. Remember: I was born in 1944. I am currently at 7 percent body fat with a resting heart rate of 40. My triglycerides are 32, my PSA is .4, and my C-reactive protein is .17. I work out two to three hours a week. I share my numbers for a couple of reasons. First, I want to prove to you that, no matter how busy you are, it is possible to achieve and sustain the truly lean body and the optimal health you want and deserve. Hopefully, you find that encouraging. Second, black-and-white, empirical, objective measurements are an integral component of The Joe Dillon Difference lifestyle. You cannot fake objective, empirical results. Your body does not lie.

As we continue to learn, we constantly fine-tune The Joe Dillon Difference lifestyle. Keep in mind, since 1979, The Joe Dillon Difference lifestyle has stood the test of time. It has been relentlessly reviewed, challenged, and practiced by thousands of people every day. And remember our mantra: First, do no harm.

Sandy Terrien's Story

I am Joe Dillon's partner in business and in life. I realize you have probably just finished reading Joe's amazing and inspirational story. I can't begin to compete with that. I did not experience nearly as dramatic a life-altering situation that inspired me to pursue my quest of health. In fact, most of my life, I thought I had a pretty good handle on nutrition and exercise. But I realize now it was just youth that gave me that illusion.

In my teens and early twenties, I really did not suffer from a weight problem, and I was always very healthy and vibrant. I never really stopped to think about my nutrition and health. Actually, I never really stopped to think about a lot of things. As I grew older, however, I began to struggle with excess weight, depression, stress, and mood swings. And I must admit it really caught me by surprise. It seemed like it happened overnight. In reality, it had been a slow and insidious process I was not aware of because I was not paying attention, and I really did not truly understand the biochemistry of the body. I had forgotten to listen to my body.

As I share my story, I am guessing you may find that many of the issues I dealt with are very similar to yours. This is why I am co-authoring this book with Joe and why my knowledge, expertise, and experiences can help you better understand how The Joe Dillon Difference lifestyle can truly have a positive, life-changing impact on your health and well-being.

Through my work with many clients, both men and women, in our one-on-one coaching program, as well as the many emails and phone calls I receive daily, I constantly hear people's stories, and I am always amazed by how similar we all are. Repeatedly, people share their frustrations with weight loss, uncontrollable mood swings, and lack of energy. So often, women especially have only fashion models and movie stars to compare ourselves to. How fair is that? For those of us who live in the real world, it can be pretty depressing. Many people feel hopeless and lost, bombarded with information that is contradictory and just doesn't work. It has become increasingly apparent to me that conventional wisdom has failed us in addressing these needs—and the growing epidemic of obesity, stress-related

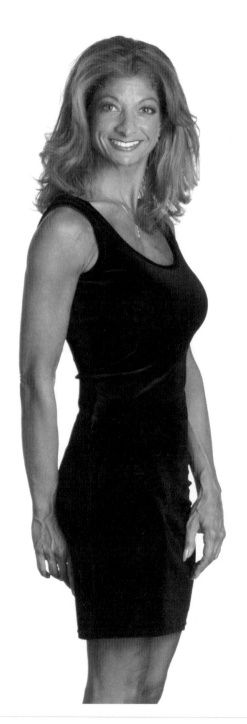

Sandy Terrien

anxiety, and depression in the population proves that. Now there is real hope; there is good, solid information that really works. Unfortunately, it took me many years to understand this difference and even more years to find Joe and his program so I had the information I needed to *really* become the lean and healthy person I am today.

Born in 1957, I grew up in Massachusetts in an upper-middle-class family. My dad was a dentist. Unfortunately, he was a dentist with a drinking problem. My mom was a stay-at-home mom who assumed that her professional husband would always take care of her. On the outside, it appeared as if we had all the comforts a family could ask for—but that was a far cry from the reality of my life. My dad was highly intelligent and an extremely skilled dentist with a good heart who loved deeply, but he suffered from extreme depression and lack of self-esteem, which manifested itself in cruelty and alcoholism. It was very sad to watch and live through this.

My mom had had a very traumatic childhood herself, and although she was quite beautiful, she too was very insecure. She entered adulthood unprepared to deal with life, never mind this very challenging situation. She did not possess the insight, nor did she have the desire to attain this insight, which would have allowed her to rise above this situation and nurture and inspire her children so they could overcome such a dysfunctional environment. In many ways, she was still a child herself, searching for the love and nurturing she never received as a child. And so there I was, trying to figure out life on my own and without the benefit of the mentoring I so needed from my parents.

I was extremely bright, excelled in school, and always received straight A's. I tried so hard to be the "dutiful daughter," eager to please, hoping to be loved, and thinking that if I did all these things, everyone would be happy and all would be right with the world. This is a very common reaction among children of alcoholics and dysfunctional families, and as this book unfolds, you will better understand how we truly are products of our past and how much influence genetics and epigenetics have over us.

So although I was proud of my academic accomplishments, I never thought about what fantastic opportunities and exciting career options this ability might bring me. In fact, I never really thought about who and what I wanted to be in life. Instead, I spent most of my time romanticizing about the "perfect" marriage, family, and life I was determined to find. What I really wanted was to be loved. Unfortunately, I didn't get that I had to love and respect myself first. I did not know how to accept myself and feel proud and good about who I was. The best education in the world cannot give you that, and unfortunately, my parents did not have the parenting skills to give me that foundation.

Even after my dad died when I was ten years old and my mom had to return to the workforce as a secretary (her only skill), I didn't get the importance of education, of having a real career, and truly being able to thrive in the world on your own two feet. Even after our standard of living declined because of her limited earning potential, I didn't get it. I squandered my intellectual talents and my superior academic achievements because, despite all of the possibilities that might have existed for me out in the world, none of it mattered. I just wanted to be a wife and mother and to find love.

This was in the late 1960s and early 1970s, when the thought of women "having it all" was just beginning. At that time, it was still common practice for women to think that their lives should revolve around the house and the family. And yes, we might be required to work outside the home if finances dictated that, but our career was never really meant to be a "career"—not one that might interfere with the responsibilities of the home anyway. Many women still feel that way today, which is fine as long as you, as a woman, do not forget that you matter too. If you make that decision, make sure you are making it for the right reasons. Unfortunately, I never got that concept.

So initially, I went to college in Boston, and then I began my career as a dental hygienist. It seemed like the perfect choice. I'm sure even the most amateurish of psychotherapists can figure out why I chose dentistry, and the reason I picked hygiene instead of going for my DDS was because I figured this "job" was just temporary. Just a way of supporting myself until the "perfect" man came along. As much as I truly enjoyed my patients and colleagues, pretty early on in my career, I began to feel stagnant and unchallenged. I knew I was meant to be something more. I knew I was selling myself short and failing to tap into my potential. Still single, and concerned that I might remain that way, I started to think about career options for the first time in my life. Since I had a passion for health and the workings of the human body, I returned to college to continue my studies in health sciences and physiology, with the intention of continuing on to graduate school. I was working full time and attending classes full time—quite an overwhelming feat, if I do say so myself. In spite of this demanding schedule, I received my bachelor's degree, graduated Summa Cum Laude with straight A's, and was very excited about my path and future. I thought I was finally coming into my own. I was on my way to graduate school, full of hope and a whole new world filled with opportunities. Then my life changed.

I fell in love and married. Unfortunately, that meant relocating with my husband and abandoning my plans for graduate school. About one and a half years later, I gave birth to a beautiful daughter. What can I say? Old habits die hard. And old dysfunctions that have not been resolved die even harder. I have absolutely no regrets about my decisions, and I have a wonderful, strong, independent, beautiful daughter, who I love more than anything. But I failed myself in so many ways when I made this decision without the proper self-examination and without having learned how to love myself first. I did not ask myself some very important questions. At the time, love and the promise of happily ever after was all I could think about. After all, that had always been my dream. I never stopped to think about how this decision would affect my life. How many doors was I closing by not continuing my education? How many wonderful opportunities would I be turning my back on? Where would this decision leave me if I was wrong and he was not the perfect man? In fact, since no person is perfect, nor can they fill the void that exists within us as individuals, shouldn't I have done the hard work of becoming all that I, as an individual, could become first? Of course I should have. But I jumped in, full speed ahead, anyway.

Before too long, the reality of marriage began to show up. Many of my husband's plans didn't work out as well as he had hoped. He was struggling with his own demons and not necessarily conquering them. I had to return to dental hygiene to help support the family. And like many men, my husband did not understand the concept of sharing the household responsibilities, despite the fact that I was working full time as well. Since I was the one who seemed to be responsible for managing our household and taking care of our daughter and family, of course there was no time left for me. As the years went by, I got more and more caught up in the Mommy-comes-last lifestyle. I had let life's responsibilities and the needs of others become more important than my life, my needs, and my health and fitness. I had moved from the dutiful daughter to the dutiful wife and mother mode. But I didn't speak up, at least not often enough or to ears that were listening.

The bottom line is that, as women, we as a rule, *allow* our needs to come last. The family and everyone else's needs come first. Women are famous for living that reality. We grow up in a culture that encourages us to be nurturers to everyone but *ourselves*. If we take time for ourselves, we feel guilty—we think we're being selfish or neglecting those who need us. But taking care of ourselves is one of the most unselfish things we can do. After all, we are the glue that holds everything together. When we fall apart, everything falls apart. When we're sad and miserable, *everyone* is sad and miserable. We put ourselves at the bottom of the priority list, and then we feel angry when no one comes to our rescue and tells us we deserve more. We need to remember that we do deserve more: We deserve to be loved and respected. But we are the ones who need to respect ourselves enough first, before we are able to command that respect from others. So again, remember that. *You* matter. *Your* needs matter.

Unfortunately, I didn't remember that. As I moved through my thirties, I started putting on weight. Since I really did not suffer from a weight problem in my teens and early twenties, I never really stopped to think about my nutrition and health, so this really caught me by surprise. Now I felt out of shape and was not exercising; I felt tired and stressed all the time; I seemed to have more downs than ups; all my passion for life seemed to be gone; and the once-vibrant, healthy person I had always been seemed to be slipping away. My lack of self-esteem, my lack of feeling important and heard, my disappointment in myself for not valuing myself enough to stand up for me and command the respect I deserved, and my anger at myself for not pursuing a more fulfilling career, began to take its toll on my life, my body, and my marriage. And I, like many, found comfort in food. For a while, I felt my weight gain and negative emotions were just something I had to accept as part of life. It was part of the cycle of getting older, one of life's cruel, but inevitable realities. I didn't realize until many years later that I was the one who could break this cycle. But as I prepared to enter my forties, I decided I didn't want to accept this any longer; I wanted my life and my health and my body back! I was determined to get myself and my life back into shape.

By this time, my husband had left our marriage, my daughter was growing up, and I felt more lost than ever. Everything that had defined me as a woman was changing, and although the status quo had certainly been less than perfect, at least I knew what the status quo was. So despite the fact that my life choices had taken their toll on my body and my self-esteem, at least they were something I could count on. Now I felt like I couldn't count on anything. I had to reinvent myself, or perhaps invent myself for the first time, and travel down that scary road of answering my own questions: "Who am I? And what do I really want out of life?"

I began that journey with my quest for a new and healthy body, a body that would go with my new life. After all, since I was a Summa Cum Laude graduate who specialized in the area of health science and physiology, I knew I was smart. I knew I had a background in science and physiology—how difficult could it be? But for whatever reason, even with all my training in biochemistry and body mechanics, figuring out how to lose weight, keep it off, and really get healthy and lean was a huge problem for me. Maybe weight loss was just too emotional an issue for me to look at it scientifically. Or maybe I just didn't realize how caught up in conventional wisdom and media hype I actually was. We get bombarded daily with pictures of movie stars, news of the newest "miracle diet," and quick-fix strategies that are "guaranteed" to work. And like many of you, I believed them. Or at least I wanted to.

So I joined a gym and started watching my diet. Anxious to see results, at first I tried all the fad diets. I tried the counting-points diet, the prepackaged-food diets, and everything else. But of course, none of them worked for very long. Eventually, I just fell into the trap of starving myself and overtraining. I started working out as hard as I could, for two and a half hours a day, because I figured when it came to exercise, harder and longer was better. Right? And I began cutting my calories as severely as I could, because I figured when it came to eating, less is better. Right?

Boy was I wrong. Between working full time, working out, and taking care of my daughter and household, I had no time for a life. Plus, I was so hungry and exhausted all the time that I was miserable and my mood swings were out of control. Oh, and then there were those cravings that would hit me between the hours of 8 or 9 PM until bedtime. It would end with either hours of pure torture or a total breakdown in which I undid all of the dietary control I had exercised during the day. I found myself with the uncontrollable need to eat all the ice cream, cookies, chocolates, or chips I could find. And I still wouldn't feel satisfied, just disgusted and depressed. It seemed that no matter what I did, I just couldn't keep the weight off. In fact, I had to keep eating less and less just not to put the weight back on.

You know what that's like, that whole yo-yo concept of dieting. We do our best, but we feel so deprived, hungry, and miserable that we just can't sustain it. And then we stop losing weight and get so frustrated that we go off our diet completely and put back on all the weight we've lost and then some. Then, of course, we blame ourselves. We feel horrible about ourselves. We call ourselves weak and a failure. And even worse, we're now fatter than we were before, so when we look in the mirror—or God forbid, we look at ourselves naked in the mirror—we're constantly reminded of exactly how much of a failure we are. And what's the answer to feeling bad about ourselves? We say, "To heck with it, I might as well eat!" It was a nightmare. I'm guessing many of you may have lived that nightmare too.

I even went back to school to become a certified personal trainer. And they did teach me a lot about weight training, which was very helpful, but they, too, seemed to be caught in this world of conventional wisdom, unable to think outside the box and really delve into the biochemistry of the body to figure out why the diet industry is a multibillion dollar industry and yet Americans keep getting fatter and fatter. So now I not only had my own goals as a motivator, but I also had clients who were looking to me for guidance. I owed it to them and myself to find those answers, to really make a difference. I started reading everything I could get my hands on. I started doing research into health and fitness and trying new things. I read everything I could on self-development and self-esteem building. I was on a mission. I was determined. I was going to figure out what I was missing.

Then I met Joe Dillon. One of Joe's favorite sayings is, "When the student is ready, the teacher will appear." Well, that certainly was the case for me. Joe taught me so much. I learned what it was to be "skinny-fat." I had cut my calories so low and overtrained so much that, even though I had lost a fair amount of weight, most of the weight I had lost was from my lean body mass (my muscles, bones, and fluids). To add to that, I had depleted my lean body mass so drastically that my metabolism had slowed to a crawl. That's why I had to keep eating less and less, just to avoid putting the weight back on.

By adopting Joe's lifestyle of proper nutrition, exercise, and supplementation, I not only regained my lean mass and got leaner, I regained my life. I reduced my workout time from two and a half hours, six to seven days a week, to forty-five minutes, four to five times per week, and I was no longer exhausted. Instead, I felt invigorated. In fact, I had more energy than I'd had in years. And since Joe's nutritional program encourages you to eat four to six times per day, I was no longer hungry all the time. I never felt deprived, and even my mood swings and cravings went away. And it wasn't just my body that was changing. Because of the nutritional changes I had made, my brain chemistry and emotional state also dramatically changed. My entire thought process and attitude toward life was more positive. My self-esteem sky-rocketed and I began to feel empowered and centered. My new body was now the external embodiment of the healthy, positive, confident inner me I had become.

One of the biggest changes I noticed was when I stopped eating processed sugar. I never realized how addicted to sugar I actually was. A common characteristic of children of alcoholics, addicts, and children of obese parents is they have a tendency to become "dry drunks." This means that although they may manage to escape the pitfalls of alcoholism or drug addiction, they are still addicts. The problem is that their drug of choice is sugar. Because sugar is legal and does not carry the stigma associated with other "drugs," their addiction usually goes unchecked—but they *are* suffering from addiction. People who are sugar addicts tend to be very sensitive to sugar and crave carbohydrates (especially refined sugar), and they use those foods for comfort as a way of coping. Sugar is one of the most addictive substances, so you can see what a harmful way of coping this can become. Unchecked, this problem leads to a host of problems like obesity, depression, mood swings, heart disease, and type 2 diabetes, to name a few. Because I suffered from this addiction, unbeknownst to me, I felt caught in this crazy cycle and could not figure out how to escape. I never realized what a powerful medication sugar actually was. The Joe Dillon Difference lifestyle finally helped me learn how to stabilize my blood sugar and eventually end my addiction to sugar and become truly healthy, inside and out.

Why is stable blood sugar so important? Because without stable blood sugar, you cannot think clearly and make rational decisions.

And why am I so sugar sensitive and how does that affect my well-being? This question has been a guiding force in our research. As Joe and I have pursued our research into the challenges most humans experience, many of the causes of my problems have become apparent to me, especially as we explored the area of fetal and childhood development. When a baby is young (and also when they are developing in the womb), the most important things they need are love, security, and healthy nutrition, so their body feels safe. They need to know these things are consistent. They need to know it is non-negotiable, that they are truly safe and can count on that throughout their life. That need may be met by a mother, father, grandparent, or any loving person, but it needs to be there. When a child grows up without these things, they find the world a scary place instead of a safe and nurturing place. Remember, to a child, home is their world. So if home is scary and unsafe, then the world must be scary and unsafe. As the child grows and ventures out into the world, they feel uncomfortable in the world and with themselves. They feel insecure about their place in the world and doubt their self-worth. Their body and their mind will be mismatched with the world. They need to fill that void with something: drugs, alcohol, compulsive shopping, gambling, promiscuity, and/or the most common medication—sugar and overeating. Although we cannot undo the damage done in our childhood it is not too late.

Quite often, we hear that we need to be our own hero, our own best friend, and I agree. However, in the past, that sentiment never really resonated with me. What does it mean to be my own hero? I just couldn't relate, and I couldn't figure out how to be that person; it felt like an empty saying to me. But now I understand.

You can still become that "loved child" and fill that void with something healthy. **Be that "loving, nurturing mother" to *yourself*. Love and nourish yourself as if you are the child you love more than anything. Be your own hero.** Love yourself unconditionally even when you make mistakes, but teach yourself to learn from those mistakes. Forgive yourself for your imperfections, but still have expectations for yourself. Tell yourself how proud you are of who you are, but never stop reaching to become even better and stronger. Be generous with your praise for yourself, but don't let yourself off the hook too easily. Expect greatness from yourself, because you are great. Fuel yourself with healthy nutrition, so your body feels its best. And remember that you deserve health and happiness. You do deserve to be loved and respected. Make choices in your life that are congruent with that message. It took me decades to figure that out (and I'm still working on it). So if these words resonate with you, pay attention to what we are about to teach you throughout this book. People with such sugar sensitivity need to be very careful with the nutrition they choose, and

The Joe Dillon Difference lifestyle is the absolute best program you will ever find to help you deal with this issue.

The reason I know this to be true is that it wasn't just me who was experiencing these remarkable changes. As the months went by, I began to see the same positive changes in the lives and bodies of my clients; it was incredible. I knew that pursuing a career in health and having a positive impact on the lives and health of people was my calling. As the saying goes, "We teach best what we most need to learn." The more I helped my clients become happy, healthy, and feel really good about themselves, the more fit I became and the better I felt about myself. I had truly found a win/win situation. I was so passionate about my new focus, and I had never felt more fulfilled. And because I was so impressed with Joe and the amazing lifestyle program he had created, I knew I couldn't ignore this opportunity. So I listened to what my inner self was saying to me for the first time in my life. Since my daughter was now in college, I decided to take a leap of faith. I quit my job, moved three thousand miles from my home in Connecticut to California, and began working with Joe. I was confident that by partnering with Joe I could reach so many more people and positively affect so many more lives.

Here it is, many years later, and I have never been happier. I have a fantastic, caring, and loving relationship with Joe. I am the mother of a beautiful daughter and a grandmother of a beautiful boy. I still work full time (although now I love my job); I still have a household to run (although Joe is a wonderful help-mate); I have tremendous business and personal obligations, and I have even successfully traveled down the road of menopause. Despite my busy life and the fact that I was born in 1957 (so I am certainly no kid), I am five feet, five inches, 106-–108 pounds, 10–12 percent body fat, a size 0–2, and I feel terrific. I feel positive, alive, sexy, and proud of who I am and what I have chosen to do with my life. And because I feel so good about myself and have actually learned to love and honor myself, I am also a better partner, lover, and mother. Again, everyone wins. Isn't that a wonderful way to live?

My presence and input have given Joe's program the added dimension of a woman's perspective. My educational background in health science and physiology, coupled with my highly developed research skills; my many years as a personal coach; and my past experiences have expanded our program to an even greater level of understanding than either of us could have

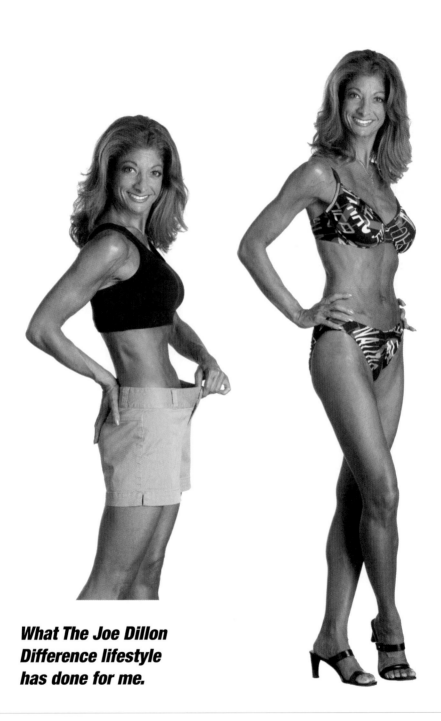

**What The Joe Dillon
Difference lifestyle
has done for me.**

reached alone. I am honored to serve as a woman's voice and as the touch-stone to the plight of women everywhere in an effort to hopefully save women (and men, if my story resonates with them) from going through the years of heartache and frustration I went through. And for those of you who have already lived my nightmare, rest assured, The Joe Dillon Difference lifestyle will give you the information and guidance you need to finally put that behind you: real hope, and good, solid, safe information that really works. Every day, I receive emails of thanks and gratitude from those who attend our seminars and are now living our lifestyle, and let me tell you, they mean more to me than I can ever express. This is why I can be so confident that health, happiness, and fitness can be an option at any age, no matter what your life is like. I am so honored to have this opportunity to share my story with you and help you become the happy, healthy, lean, and sexy person you know you deserve to be.

Section One

Major Challenges to Weight Loss

Chapter 1

The Evolutionary Challenge

Evolutionary science is the fundamental organizing principle
of all biology.
—Peter Gluckman, MD, Alan Beedle, MD, and Mark
Hanson, MD, *Principles of Evolutionary Medicine*, 2010

In the middle of the nineteenth century, Charles Darwin (1809–1882) had one of the most profound insights in all of human history: evolution. Darwin's first book, *The Origin of Species*, was published in 1859. Darwin's book sold out immediately and created a firestorm of controversy. Darwin's insights changed our understanding of biology forever. At nearly the same time, Gregor Mendel (1822–1884) had some profound insights into genetics. Mendel's one and only paper, *Experiments in Plant Hybridization*, was published in 1865. Unlike Darwin's instant fame, Mendel's work went basically unnoticed for more than thirty years. Neither Darwin nor Mendel was aware of the other's work. Yet just as Darwin is considered the father of evolutionary science, Mendel is considered the father of modern genetics. It is within the context of the work of Darwin (and modern evolutionary biology) and Mendel (and modern, high-tech genetics) that we will view the challenge of losing weight.

Today, because of the sequencing of the human genome (completed in 2003), our understanding of genetics in general and our own human genetics in particular is growing by leaps and bounds. Modern genetics has also shed considerable light on human evolution through insights provided by mitochondrial DNA and Y-chromosome testing. We can now trace our genetic heritage as *Homo sapiens* all the way back to Africa. In light of our new and better understanding of evolution, genes, and genetics, we feel it might be helpful to share a few insights about genes. The human genome includes about three billon genes. Even though only about twenty-five thousand of your genes are supposedly "active," it turns out to be much more complicated than that. Many of the supposedly "inactive" genes turn out to be actively involved in the regulation of the "active" genes. Genes do not turn themselves on or off. It takes a specialized protein messenger molecule to turn on any particular gene. Gene expression also dictates what kind of cell will develop. All cells in your body contain your complete genome—in other words, your entire genetic inheritance is coded into every cell. Yet selective gene expression means that only certain genes will be expressed in any particular cell, and this pattern of expression determines what kind of cell it will be. Heart cells are heart cells because of gene expression. The same goes for liver cells, kidney cells, and brain cells. Each is coded in a particular way.

This range in gene expression is responsible for the incredible diversity among humans—even though, statistically speaking, there is less than one-half of 1 percent genetic difference between any two human beings on earth. This immense variety among human beings underscores the huge range of expression possible with basically the same set of genes. The point is simple: Your genetic inheritance is *not* etched in stone.

We find it easiest to think of genetic inheritance as a set of strategies or biological tendencies. It is not absolute. Just because someone in your family had a metabolic disorder like diabetes, obesity, or heart disease doesn't mean you are going to have that problem. All it means is that you may be more susceptible or vulnerable to that same issue. How you developed (fetal programming) and your current lifestyle as an adult also have a big impact.

Human beings are extremely complex organisms. Individual genes are made up of base pairs of amino acids bonded by a hydrogen molecule. These base pairs are wound up in the famous double-helix shape of DNA. A single gene may include more than one thousand base pairs. Yet it is extremely rare (less than one tenth of 1 percent) for any single gene to control any given human trait. In 99.9 percent of traits, dozens to hundreds of genes working together control traits. You can begin to see the profound level of complexity of your body and the impact of your genetic inheritance.

Unfortunately, popular media gives the false and totally misleading impression that one gene equals one trait. We hear in the media all the time how science has discovered "the" gene for a given trait, such as "the" cancer gene. By vastly oversimplifying genetic complexity, the popular media raises false hopes in the general public. In reality, the interaction between a person's genome (their inherited genetic material), his or her development (epigenetics), his or her lifestyle, and the environment is a mind-boggling, extremely complex dynamic and changes throughout a lifetime.

It's also important to understand how far back in history your genome extends. Every human being carries billions of years of evolutionary history inside every single cell in their body. This is the science of evolutionary biology. As we take you through this chapter, and you start to wonder, "Why do I have to know all of this stuff about evolution?" please bear with us. We promise you will see why understanding how human beings evolved is so crucial if you want to overcome the challenges we face in trying to win at the game of weight loss.

The Evolution of a Species

The purpose of this chapter is to establish the evolutionary perspective from which or through which weight loss is viewed. The perspective of evolutionary biology is like putting on a special set of glasses. These special glasses will enable you to see clearly (maybe for the very first time) the biological reality of your body and the multiple challenges you face when trying to lose weight. The fact is each of us is dealt a certain hand in life. These cards are what we have to work with, so the better you understand the game, as well as the assets and liabilities of the cards you are holding, the more effectively you can play the game of weight loss. Metaphorically speaking, the most fundamental cards in your hand are evolution and your DNA (your genome). With this perspective: What is the nature of your evolutionary-genetic challenge when it comes to trying to lose weight?

To begin at the very beginning, our earth was formed roughly 4.6 billion years ago. It took about five hundred million more years for the hydrosphere to stabilize, which means our planet became watery about four billion years ago. Without water, there would be no life on earth. About this same time, prebiotic (pre-life) organic chemistry developed in the form of a primordial soup of organic molecules. No life had formed yet, but the fundamental building blocks of life (organic protein molecules) were present. This was a pre-RNA world. Pre-RNA molecules were the building blocks of our earliest genetic material. They were a way to communicate genetic information.

For life to exist on our planet, two criteria had to be met:

- **First, the organism must survive.**

- **Second, the organism must have a way to communicate the "recipe" to replicate, some way to communicate genetic information.**

By 3.8 billion years ago, earth had transformed from a pre-RNA world to an RNA world. These RNA molecules were self-replicating organic molecules. They were the earliest genetic material that was able to duplicate itself. RNA molecules were the ancient precursors for DNA. But the RNA molecules reproduced themselves with no intrinsic variation. Each one was exactly the same. Their replication also required resources that were limited, such as energy, space, and smaller organic building blocks. Limited resources resulted in Darwinian competition. According to Darwin's theory of evolution, natural selection favored molecules that are more efficient and more effective at reproducing themselves in a given environment.

Around 3.6 billion years ago, the first DNA molecules and protein life appeared. The DNA molecule reproduced itself more efficiently and more effectively than the RNA molecule. As a result, DNA molecules took over as the main replicators. Why? Because DNA molecules were fitter; that is, DNA molecules reproduced more effectively.

These archaic genomes soon developed bilayer membranes that enclosed the molecule and provided a more stable environment for replication. These were the first proto-cells, or precursors to true cells. The earliest version of the DNA molecule found in every single cell in your body evolved about 3.6 billion years ago (Barton et al. 2007).

Approximately 3.5 billion years ago, the first *true* simple cells appeared. At this time, the primitive atmosphere had virtually no oxygen. The earliest atmosphere was composed of methane, ammonia, hydrogen, and water. As a result, the very earliest single cell organisms were all anaerobic. Anaerobic means that their metabolisms did not need oxygen.

Some of these simple cells were photosynthesizing cyanobacteria, which used carbon dioxide as a carbon source and oxidized inorganic materials to extract energy. Photosynthesis is the process that captures energy from the sun and converts that energy into chemical energy. All plants use photosynthesis, and life on our planet could not exist without photosynthesis. Cyanobacteria used water as a reducing agent and produced oxygen as a waste product. Over time, the oxygen concentration in our earth's atmosphere began to rise.

These simple single-celled organisms are called prokaryotes. Prokaryotic cells are basically simple double-membraned bags of saline (salty) water with some genetic material (DNA) floating around inside. Today's bacteria are examples of prokaryotic cells. Later, prokaryotes evolved to carry out glycolysis. Glycolysis is a set of chemical reactions that frees organic molecules such as glucose, and stores their released energy in chemical bonds of ATP (adenosine triphosphate). In simple terms, glycolysis means the metabolism of sugar. Your brain and body are burning glucose and ATP as you read these words. In fact, every single cell in your entire body is using thousands of ATP molecules per second as energy. Glycolysis and ATP continue to be used in almost every cell of every animal (including human beings) to this day, billions of years after the first cells developed this adaptation.

This is consistent with evolutionary theory. Evolution is both conservative and cumulative. When evolution finds something that works, it builds upon it until something is developed that is more fit, that is, that works even better in a given environment. Replication and metabolism are key properties of life.

Around 1.85 billion years ago, eukaryotic cells appeared. All the cells in every animal (including every cell in our bodies) are eukaryotic cells. Eukaryotic cells are highly complex cells that contain membrane-bound organelles (cell components) such as a nucleus, which is where your DNA is located. Eukaryotic cells also contain mitochondria. Mitochondria are the energy producing organelles in cells. They continuously produce energy in the form of ATP—even as you're reading these words. These complex cells and their organelles are protected by membranes made from essential fats. The membrane's job is complex: It allows for the passage of materials and water into and out of the cell's interior and protects the cell.

This was the very beginning of homeostasis. Homeostasis is a dynamic process that attempts to keep your interior milieu stable and constant. Our relatively constant body temperature is a classic example of homeostasis. The temperature set-point for most human beings is 98.6 degrees Fahrenheit (plus or minus). If you get too hot, you sweat to cool yourself off. If you get too cold, you shiver to generate heat to warm yourself back up. These responses are examples of homeostasis at work.

Approximately 1.2 billion years ago, sexual reproduction appeared. Sexual reproduction significantly accelerated the rate of evolution. Why? Because each time you have sexual reproduction, you have a new combination of genetic information: half from the mother and half from the father. Sexual reproduction gave evolution and natural selection dramatically more material to work with to find the fittest organisms. Sexual reproduction gave organisms a more effective, faster way to adapt to changing environments.

About the same time (1.2 billion years ago), simple multicellular organisms evolved. These earliest multicellular organisms mostly consisted of cell colonies with limited complexity.

From approximately 700 million years ago to 540 million years ago, a second major increase in the oxygen content of our earth's atmosphere took place. Since enough oxygen had accumulated in the atmosphere, this allowed the formation of an ozone layer. The ozone layer blocked enough solar radiation to permit the first colonization of the land. Somewhere between 580 and 540 million years ago, the first large, complex, multicellular organisms appeared. Thus, it took about four billion years from the formation of the earth for the very first truly complex multicellular life forms to appear.

Now things really began to speed up (at least on an evolutionary time scale). Approximately 540 million years ago, the Cambrian Explosion took place. The first known footprints on land by amphibians appeared 530 million years ago; the first vertebrates appeared 485 million years ago; the first footprints by land animals appeared 395 million years ago.

The oxygen content of our earth's atmosphere continued to rise, until it peaked at about 35 percent about three hundred million years ago. There was so much oxygen and the atmosphere of our earth was so dense, it enabled the growth of huge insects. For example, dragonflies had wing spans of 2.5 feet. Eventually, the atmosphere settled back down to approximately 21 percent oxygen, as it is today.

Two hundred twenty-five million years ago, the earliest dinosaurs appeared; the earliest mammals appeared 215 million years ago. As you know, we human beings are mammals. Now you can see how essential oxygen is to the existence of life and why we consider oxygen number one when it comes to the biological essentials of life.

Approximately 65 million years ago, a major extinction event took place that eliminated half of all the animal species on the earth, including all the dinosaurs. Over the next 30 million years, mammals became the dominant species for the first time. Thirty-five million years ago, many modern mammal groups began to appear, including dogs, sloths, and eagles.

Twenty-five million years ago, a very early primate called Proconsul appeared. Proconsul is considered a possible ancestor to both lesser and greater apes and to humans. Fifteen million years ago, great apes speciated (diverged or split-off) from ancestors of the gibbon (lesser apes). Ten million years ago, Hominini (our human ancestors) split-off from the ancestors of gorillas. Seven million years ago, Hominina split-off from the ancestors of chimpanzees. The earliest known human ancestor after the separation of the human and chimpanzee lines appeared approximately 6–7 million years ago.

Six million years ago, our earliest ancestors were small (about three feet tall), lived in trees, and ate mostly fruit. Aside from the occasional insect, they were vegetarians. Two major differences separated our earliest ancestors from the common ancestor they shared with chimpanzees. First, our earliest ancestors were bipedal, meaning they walked on two legs. They were bipedal apes, although they were not yet of the genus Homo as in *Homo sapiens*. They had short legs and resembled an amalgam of ape and very primitive human. They could walk fairly well on two legs (unlike the four-legged knuckle-walk of chimpanzees), but our earliest ancestors' upper bodies still enabled them to climb trees proficiently. They had brains about the size of an orange, not much bigger than the brain of a chimpanzee (Potts and Sloan 2010). They also had small canine teeth, which meant they were less intimidating to each other. This enhanced a crucial aspect of being human: more complex social interactions.

In 1974, in Hadar, Ethiopia, Donald Johanson discovered one of the most complete skeletons of our human ancestors ever found (Johanson 1981, 1989, 1996, 1999, 2009). Dr. Johanson named her "Lucy". Lucy was 3.18 million years old. Her skeleton clearly proved she walked on two legs (was bipedal). Lucy was three and half feet tall and a vegetarian. Lucy was a member of the species *Australopithecus afarensis*. The suffix "pithecus" means ape.

Five years later, in 1979, Mary Leakey made an amazing discovery. Dr. Leakey found a series of 3.7 million-year-old footprints preserved in fossilized volcanic ash and made by the same species of human ancestor as Lucy, *Australopithecus afarensis*. The footprints revealed two early human ancestors walking side by side, further strengthening the theory of increased socialization among the species and the fact they were bipedal. Mary Leakey found the footprints in Laetoli, Tanzania.

The next big evolutionary leap forward came about 2.6 million years ago when our ancient ancestors first made tools. Granted, these tools were very crude, but they were effective. By striking one rock against another, our early ancestors created rocks with sharp edges. These sharp-edged rocks allowed our early ancestors to butcher carcasses deserted by predators. These sharpened rocks marked the birth of human technology.

What were the benefits of our ancestors being able to butcher a carcass deserted by a predator? Up to this point in time, our ancestors ate a predominantly vegetarian diet with occasional small amounts of meat from small animals like rodents. They were scavenger opportunists, not hunters. After the invention of tools, they became more aggressive scavengers, meaning they banded together and drove predators off their kill. This was called power scavenging (Bunn 2005).

Getting access to and being able to butcher a carcass enabled our early ancestors to eat a steady supply of meat and fat for the first time. These are the most nutrient- and calorie-dense foods we can eat. The principle component of meat, especially the wild meat our early ancestors were beginning to eat, is complete protein. For humans, there is only one thing on earth that effectively builds muscles, bones, heart muscle, and brain: protein. Wild game also contains high amounts of all eight essential amino acids.

Wild game likewise contains very little fat, but a large percentage of the fat it does contain is omega-3, the most important essential fat. As a result, when our early ancestors ate these carcasses, they ate everything, including the brain and all the other organs. They smashed the animal's bones with rocks and ate the bone marrow. Brain and bone marrow are high in fat and especially rich in omega-3 essential fat. Along with protein, omega-3 fat is brain food.

As a result of their new high-protein, high-fat, nutrient-rich diet, our early ancestors went through several major changes. By 1.8 million years ago (roughly 800,000 years after the invention of tools and the consistent inclusion of meat and fat in the Paleolithic diet), our early ancestors' brains had grown from the size of an orange to the size of a grapefruit (Potts and Sloan 2010). Their bodies had grown bigger and taller (over six feet tall). With their longer legs, our early ancestors could cover miles of ground every day, hunting and foraging. Their maximum lifespan began to increase from about twenty-five years to fifty to sixty years.

Granted, most Paleolithic people did not live long—but not because they were unhealthy. Paleolithic hunter-gatherers were exceptionally healthy, with no obesity and none of the metabolic degenerative diseases that plague modern humans.

However, Paleolithic hunter-gatherers faced real, tangible, and immediate dangers. First and foremost, they faced the constant challenge of the uncertainty of food acquisition. Paleolithic hunter-gatherers did not find a carcass every day. Because of the uncertainty of their food supply, our early ancestors evolved to easily store fat as a buffer against the uncertainty of food acquisition. They gorged themselves on meat and fat whenever there was an abundance of food, such as when they found or killed a large animal.

Their world itself also posed numerous threats, including predation by other animals such as large cats. Our early ancestors were a favorite meal for leopards. There was also the constant threat of infection, which often led to an early death. With no soap and water or wonder drugs, any wound that got infected was life-threatening. I personally experienced this while in combat in the jungles of South Vietnam. I spent weeks without a shower or even soap and water, and any little cut or scratch got infected and stayed infected. These infections sometimes lasted for months. I still have the scars from some of those infected sores all over my legs. Our early ancestors never got the opportunity to wash with soap and water, so infections just kept getting worse. But with their growing brains and with their ever-more-complex social interactions, our early ancestors were becoming better and better adapted. Adaptability is one of the hallmarks of what it means to be human.

Some people object to the idea that Paleolithic humans were intrinsically healthier than modern humans. They claim that if Paleolithic humans had lived as long as we do, they would have all the degenerative diseases we have. An obvious answer to this objection is the fact that we now have eight-year-olds with type 2 diabetes. And we have hunter-gatherers in the world today who live to be over one hundred years of age with none of the modern degenerative diseases (Lindeberg 2010).

Evidence of another major milestone in human evolution appeared about eight hundred thousand years ago: Humans learned to control and use fire. The control of fire further enhanced early humans' diet with the advent of cooking. Cooking made food both more palatable and more digestible. Paleolithic humans cooked their meat as well as the tubers they dug out of the ground.

About five hundred thousand years ago, our ancestors' brains went through a final growth spurt to our current size: about the size of a cantaloupe (Potts and Sloan 2010). It's sometimes said that human beings have the largest brains of any animal on earth. This is not true. We have the largest brains relative to our body size. This makes human beings the most intelligent organisms on the planet.

Also about this time, around four hundred thousand years ago, the first signs of more sophisticated tools and hunting weapons began to appear in the fossil record. Our ancestors no longer had to rely on scavenging for a consistent supply of meat and fat. Wooden spears skillfully shaped like javelins enabled our ancestors to become effective hunters. Paleolithic hunters began to kill more and bigger animals. Bones of large-hoofed animals and even elephants with the clear-cut marks of butchery show up at the hearths of this time period. The tools these early humans made showed greater sophistication and sharper, more precise cutting blades. Paleolithic humans soon began to attach these extremely sharp points to the ends of their throwing spears to create lethal killing tools.

About two hundred fifty thousand years ago, another major milestone appeared: the first signs of symbolic thought. The earliest artifacts were in the form of simple body ornaments. Signs of the use of ocher (a rich red color) to decorate their bodies also appeared.

Our own species, *Homo sapiens,* first appeared on the earth approximately two hundred thousand years ago. It is important to remember where anatomically modern humans first showed up. True *Homo sapiens* first appeared on the African savanna in East Africa. The earliest known fossils of anatomically modern humans were found in Ethiopia. We humans had evolved in eastern, central, and southern Africa over a span of six to seven million years through major climate changes including severe droughts. Paleolithic human beings, the first *Homo sapiens*, were hunter-gatherers who lived in small bands of twenty to thirty people. The majority of their diet (70–80 percent meat and fat) came from wild game, which they killed with the hard physical exercise of ever-more-efficient hunting (Stanford and Bunn 2001; Zimmer 2005; Ungar 2007). Wild game supplied our ancestors with a high-protein, moderate-fat, low-carbohydrate diet that was rich in micronutrients (vitamins and minerals). Highly accurate and precise isotope studies of Paleolithic bones show no sign of any nutrient deficiencies of any kind (unlike many modern humans today).

The balance of our ancestors' diet consisted of low glycemic load carbohydrates (only about 20 percent), which were consumed in the form of totally unprocessed fruits, vegetables, and tubers that our ancestors dug up from the ground with sharpened wooden sticks and hard physical work (Liu et al 2000). And of course, the only liquid our ancestors had to drink was water. The Paleolithic lifestyle was physically demanding and uncertain. Scarcity was a constant challenge. Our Upper Paleolithic ancestors (those *Homo sapiens* who lived from 200,000 to 10,500 years ago) were lean and muscular, with tremendous endurance and vitality. Our ancestors did not suffer from any of the metabolic degenerative diseases so common today, such as diabetes, obesity, or heart disease.

Modern Humans Emerge:
The Age of Agriculture

About forty thousand years ago, there was another surge forward. Around this time, beautiful and highly sophisticated cave paintings and carved figurines begin to appear in excavation sites. Overwhelming evidence makes it clear that our ancestors by this time had evolved elaborate cultures and sophisticated communication. They developed language.

Between ten thousand and twelve thousand years ago, the agricultural revolution, or Neolithic era, began. This was the next radical change. Simultaneously, at four or five different places in the Middle East, our ancestors slowly began to cultivate cereal grains and domesticate animals. Grains are highly concentrated carbohydrates with a heavy glycemic load, meaning they significantly raise insulin. Insulin is the most powerful fat-storing hormone in the human body. Anything that dramatically raises insulin will make you fat. Cereal grains (grass seeds) were never a part of the ancestral diet (Lindeberg 2010).

With the agricultural revolution, concentrated carbohydrates in the form of cereal grains became the new foundation of the human diet, instead of meat and fat. For the first time in all of human history thus far, human beings began to consistently overeat carbohydrates. Our ancestors had evolved over literally millions of years on a high-protein, moderate-fat, low-carbohydrate diet. What carbohydrates early humans did eat in the ancestral, pre-agricultural diet were totally unprocessed. As a result, our ancestors evolved to make the most efficient use of scarce carbohydrates. With agriculture, however, humans began to eat large amounts of carbohydrates for the first time.

During the 2.5 million years that passed between the invention of the first tools and the dawn of the agricultural revolution, the human gut became smaller and shorter. We lost the big, long gut of a vegetarian ape and developed a shorter gut more like a carnivore (a meat eater). Food passes through our bodies in twenty-four hours or less. Gorillas have big guts and a long intestinal track to digest the tough, vegetarian, high-fiber food they eat. It may take a week or ten days for food to pass through the gut of a gorilla. Thus began the evolutionary clash between our bodies, which had evolved to thrive on a diet of high-protein, moderate-fat, and low-carbohydrates, and the new agricultural carbohydrate-based diet with very little meat and fat. The result: Human beings began to get fat and experience metabolic diseases of civilization, like diabetes and obesity, for the first time in all of human history. There was a genetic mismatch between the programming of millions of years of evolution and the ecological niche (an agricultural environment with a diet of predominantly cereal grains) we humans found ourselves in (Gluckman and Hanson 2008).

To compound the problem, a diet based on cereal grains also allowed agricultural humans to acquire more calories with less effort. Farmers began to grind their cereal grains into flour—thus making the carbohydrates (sugars) even more readily available. Agricultural humans no longer had to walk for miles each day hunting for meat or searching for tubers to dig up. Agricultural humans were now getting less protein to support growth. Instead, agricultural humans were eating a diet of concentrated, high glycemic load carbohydrates that stimulated the release of excessive amounts of insulin and, therefore, encouraged elevation of triglycerides and the deposit of fat in adipose tissue. The result? Human beings, who had evolved to over six feet tall, began to grow shorter. Interestingly, people who continued to live the hunter-gatherer lifestyle and eat the ancestral (Paleolithic) diet into the twentieth century never suffered any of the metabolic diseases that plague modern, urbanized humans.

With the growing agricultural revolution, human beings stayed in one place instead of following migrating game animals or harvesting seasonal fruit. As a result, human beings experienced famines for the first time in human history. Agricultural humans also built shelters. The formerly small bands of hunter-gatherers grew into bigger and bigger groups, until there began to appear villages of several hundred people. Early agricultural humans slowly began to domesticate animals. Ever larger and denser communities of farming people now lived in close proximity with newly domesticated animals.

As a result, a number of diseases showed up that agricultural humans caught from the animals they lived in close proximity with. The diseases, such as influenza, small pox, and measles, spread from the animals to the people. And then, due to population density, these diseases quickly spread among the people. For the first time, communicable diseases appeared that infected large numbers of people at the same time. This was unprecedented in human history.

Compounding this was sanitation, or rather, the lack of sanitation. With denser concentrations of both humans and domesticated animals came the growing problem of both human and animal waste. As hunter-gatherers, our ancestors were constantly moving, and the accumulation of human waste was never an issue. But with growing settlements of hundreds of people densely packed together, the issue of human and animal waste became a major issue. As the environment of a settlement became more toxic, it only exacerbated the growing problem of disease.

Also, hunter-gatherer groups were largely egalitarian. Share and share alike. Social cooperation was a major factor in the survival of early humans. There was some division of labor. Women assumed the largest part of the child-rearing responsibilities. Women also did most of the foraging for the hunter-gatherer group, gathering nuts, seeds, and fruit, and digging up tubers. Men did most of the hunting for meat and fat, which they brought back to the camp fire and shared with the group. With the advent of the agricultural revolution, this all changed.

As early agricultural settlements grew ever larger, people began to specialize. Most were involved in farming—raising crops and tending animals—but some became craftsmen who made clothes, metal tools, and weapons. Still others became warriors to protect their village, town, or later, city-state. Power structures began to emerge, as well as social hierarchies: the rich and the poor, the haves and the have-nots. And with greater population density, power structures, and growing inequalities came stress. Stress is a major contributor to excess body fat.

The End Result

Human beings evolved over six to seven million years from short, small-brained pre-humans who walked bipedally on short legs, lived in trees, and ate fruit into tall, big-brained *Homo sapiens* with long legs who walked miles a day, efficiently hunted and killed large animals, and ate a diet high in protein and fat cooked over a fire. These small egalitarian bands of hunter-gatherers were lean and healthy; they thrived despite the uncertainty of the African savanna.

With the advent of agriculture, humans suddenly (in an evolutionary sense) encountered a profound mismatch. The new, high-carbohydrate diet turned our genetic advantages into liabilities. We began to live in larger numbers, exposing us to human and animal waste and communicable diseases we were not genetically prepared for. Additionally, we were unprepared for the emergence of a social hierarchy and the climate of competition.

As a result, agricultural humans reacted to their nutritionally poor diet, with its lack of protein and fat, by growing smaller and shorter. Some agricultural humans began to get fat and stay fat for the first time in human history. Agricultural humans began to suffer from communicable diseases that infected and killed large numbers of people. And degenerative metabolic diseases such as diabetes, hypertension, and heart disease, began to appear.

Of course, the appearance of agriculture had some advantages. Growing specialization led to an explosion of technology. After a few thousand years, written language appeared, exponentially accelerating the transmission of information and knowledge. More people could learn faster. Culture and social interactions such as trade, flourished. But from a health and body fat perspective, the agricultural revolution presented human beings with an unprecedented challenge, a clash between our evolutionary-genetic predisposition (our DNA, our genome) and the growth of civilization and culture. This challenge has only become more daunting over time.

Does this mean you are doomed if you have overweight tendencies in your family? The short answer is no. Your body is a complex organism. And though your evolutionary/genetic inheritance is a deep and powerful force, it is only one of many factors influencing your body and metabolism. The most prudent advice is this: If you have overweight members in your family, the best strategy is to live a healthy lifestyle. All each of us can do is to play the cards we were dealt by life to the best of our ability. We will teach you exactly how to best play these cards through a prudent diet based on our ancestors' diet, effective exercise, and pharmaceutical-grade supplementation.

Chapter 2

The Developmental Challenge

*The universal environmental responsiveness of organisms, alongside
genes, influences individual development and organic evolution,
and this realization compels us to reexamine the major themes of
evolutionary biology in a new light.*
—Mary Jane West-Eberhard, PhD,
Developmental Plasticity and Evolution, 2003

We all carry deep history in our DNA going back literally billions of years. This history dictates certain aspects of our physiology, such as the absolute need to breathe oxygen and drink water. Human beings evolved 6–7 million years ago to thrive by being lean, physically active, and by eating a diet high in protein, moderate in fat, and low in low glycemic load, unprocessed carbohydrates.

In this chapter, you will learn that each of us also has more recent programming. These tendencies or susceptibilities are as recent as your grandmother's generation. Who you are today is called your *phenotype*. Phenotype means the expression of your genotype (your genetic inheritance). In this chapter, you will learn:

■   **How your genes interact with your environment**

- **When your genes interact with your environment**
- **Why your genes interact with your environment**
- **The short-term and long-term consequences of your genes interacting with your environment**

This gene-environment interaction is called *developmental plasticity*. Developmental plasticity refers to the fact that we are capable of forming characteristics that are well adapted to the environments in which we are likely to live (our epigenetics). In adverse circumstances, small size (low birth weight) and a slower metabolism can facilitate survival. On the other hand, larger size and a faster metabolism have reproductive advantages when resources are more abundant. These characteristics are induced in utero and during early childhood, and are even set by cues to which your parents, or even your grandparents, were exposed. Individuals developmentally adapted to one environment may be at risk when exposed to another environment when they get older.

Evidence from evolutionary and developmental biology helps us understand human development and our susceptibility to disease. Responsiveness to our mother's condition before birth prepares us so we are better suited to the environment forecasted by the cues available in utero and during early childhood. The study of the way our gene expression responds to these cues is called epigenetics. It is important to note that epigenetics has to do with the *expression* of your genetic inheritance—it does not change your genes.

To set the stage for this chapter about development, keep in mind that evolution via natural selection chooses those organisms that are both most fit (that is, best adapted to their current environment) and most adaptable (that is, the most flexible and adjustable to changes in their environment).

Developmental Plasticity in the Real World

To introduce the concept of developmental plasticity, let me start with a classic example. The British began colonizing Australia in the eighteenth and nineteenth centuries. These British colonists did everything they could to make their new home (Australia) as much like their old home (England) as possible. The one food source they could not do without were rabbits. So in 1859, twenty-four wild rabbits from the English countryside were introduced into Australia. These wild English rabbits had few natural predators in Australia and little competition for food. As a result, they reproduced so rapidly they literally became pests.

The original stock of twenty-four wild English rabbits were all genetically identical. However, Australian rabbits are now very diverse in appearance; descendants of these wild English rabbits vary in size, shape, body-fat content, coat color, and even enzyme biochemistry. The rabbits born in the hotter and more arid parts of Australia have less body fat than those rabbits living in the cooler regions. In addition, the rabbits in the hotter parts of the country developed bigger, longer ears with more blood flow to their ears. Their bigger ears help them to cool themselves more efficiently.

How does the introduction of twenty-four wild English rabbits into Australia illustrate developmental plasticity? With no changes to their original genetics, these wild English rabbits adapted so they were more fit (better suited) for all the variations of the new environments they interacted with in Australia. And these adaptations were transmitted down through generations of rabbits via epigenetic mechanisms that silenced or activated certain genes to create a variety of expressions of the original English rabbit genome.

The story of Charles Darwin's finches is another example of developmental plasticity. Darwin took a five-year voyage (1831–1836) as a naturalist around the world on the sailing ship *HMS Beagle*. On this voyage, he observed, took notes, and collected species. One of his stops included the Galapagos Islands. While in the Galapagos, Darwin collected lots of different birds. He thought they were all different species. It was not until he got home and took his bird samples to the natural history museum in London that he was told all these birds were the same species: finches.

What had happened? The same species of finch had been isolated on various islands in the chain of Galapagos Islands. Each group of finches had adapted over time to the environment on each of these islands. The clearest evidence of these adaptations to different food sources was the change in the finches' beaks. Some finches developed small, thin beaks to eat small, soft seeds on its particular island. Other finches developed big, heavy beaks to better eat bigger, tougher, harder seeds on its particular island.

These changes in the same genetic species are examples of developmental plasticity, or the variety of gene expression in the same genetic inheritance. All these changes in the finches' beaks came about as a result of a single set of genes interacting with a variety of environments. This wide variety of phenotypes (expressions of the same genotype) in the same species was a major catalyst to Darwin's thinking and to his most profound insight: Evolution by natural selection (Darwin 1859).

What do rabbits in Australia and finches in the Galapagos Islands have to do with losing weight? Each of us, as it turns out, goes through a process similar to what the rabbits and finches went through.

History of Developmental Plasticity and the Developmental Origins of Metabolic Issues

In the early to mid-1980s, an English epidemiologist named David Barker, MD, PhD, was doing research on heart disease. As he looked at the records of all the counties of England, a startling pattern leaped out at him. Despite the conventional wisdom that heart disease was a disease of affluence, Barker noticed that in the poorest counties in England, the heart disease rate was double the normal rate. This made no sense to Dr. Barker, so he began to investigate. After months of intensive research, a stunning biomarker emerged. Low birth weight babies had twice the heart disease in middle age and older than did normal weight babies. Again, this made no sense to Dr. Barker. So he began to dig even deeper. He was looking for a county or counties that had years of accurate birth weights. After months of intensive research, he found what he was looking for in the county of Hertfordshire. Barker found the largest set of records in Hertfordshire; ledgers had been maintained from 1911 to 1945 on approximately sixteen thousand men and women. These records contained birth weight, weight at one year of age, and whether the baby was weaned at one year.

The records showed that for men and women, the risk of death by heart disease was doubled in individuals born with a weight of less than 5.5 pounds. In fact, there was a continuum of changed risk across all birth weights. The risk was greatest for babies born weighing 5.5 pounds or less and decreased up to 9.5 pounds, which had the least risk. The risk began to increase again for babies born with a birth weight in excess of 9.5 pounds.

As Dr. Barker continued his research, he discovered that not only did the risk for heart disease double, but so did the risk for a number of metabolic diseases such as obesity, diabetes, hypertension, high blood lipids, and metabolic syndrome. Only those who remained lean throughout their lives escaped their programmed fate.

In Finland, Dr. Barker collaborated with Dr. Johan Eriksson and his colleagues at the National Public Health Institute in Finland. The Helsinki Birth Cohort comprises twenty thousand men and women who were born in Helsinki between 1924 and 1944. Each person had detailed information collected on their size at birth and growth throughout childhood. Their illnesses were documented. These studies in Finland have produced over ninety published papers. They showed that the increased risk of coronary heart disease, type 2 diabetes, hypertension, and stroke among people who were born small at birth was modified or amplified by the way they grew as children.

Over the last twenty years, studies in the USA, France, Holland, India, China, Thailand, and Saudi Arabia have confirmed Dr. Barker's original findings about the impact of the maternal environment and the early years of childhood on the health of people in middle and old age.

Developmental Responses to Environmental Influences

The development of an individual depends on both genes and environment. The interaction between the developing individual and environment is critical. At each phase of development, the organism may be sensitive to particular environmental cues. The effects of these responses impact subsequent stages of development. Such interactions affect many physiological systems, such as appetite, cardiovascular health, and responses to stress—each of which may confer some survival advantage in the appropriate environment.

Developmentally disruptive events irreversibly interfere with embryonic development and, depending on their nature, may have deleterious effects either in utero and/or after birth. Generally, such cues act by interfering with a developmental process during periods of vulnerability.

For example, the availability of oxygen to the fetus may be limited by the capacity of the placenta to transfer oxygen, and the fetus has no mechanism by which to increase oxygen availability. Therefore, under low oxygen conditions, the fetus must conserve oxygen by redistributing blood flow to vital organs such as the heart and brain, at the expense of others such as muscle, gut, and kidney, and by reducing oxidative metabolism. This illustrates adaptive responses made by the developing fetus that have a clear, immediate effect in utero or in the infant period.

Some responses made by the developing organism to environmental conditions may not have an immediate adaptive effect, but may manifest later in life. It needs to be emphasized that these are not simply the effects of constraint in utero, but rather mechanisms by which the fetus uses an early environmental cue to "predict its future" and adopts a developmental pathway that might best suit it to its expected postnatal or adult environment.

The efficacy of this sort of strategy depends on whether the prediction is correct (well-matched to actual environmental conditions in later life) or not (Bateson et al 2004; Gluckman and Hanson 2004). When a match between the predicted and actual environment occurs, the offspring will thrive. When the prediction is incorrect, however, the organism is left with a postnatal physiology that is mismatched and inappropriate, putting it at increased risk for weight gain and disease (Gluckman and Hanson 2004). So whether this "cue" becomes a benefit or a liability will depend on a number of features: the accuracy of the cue and the various environmental states, as well as the consequences of the mismatch (Gluckman and Hanson 2004). Such errors in prediction might arise either because the postnatal environment has shifted or because the fetus has received faulty information on which to base its prediction.

Coping and Tradeoffs

Between the pathological and adaptive extremes, the developing organism might be forced by environmental exposure to "cope" in ways that might involve homeostatic mechanisms or substantial adjustments in physiology and morphology to ensure survival. Sometimes this coping has long-term effects on Darwinian fitness by imposing costs that impact the individual at a later stage in its life. For example, a general fetal response to maternal nutritional deprivation is to reduce fetal growth (Harding and Gluckman 2001). The fetus cannot outgrow the supply of nutrients delivered across the placenta, and matching growth to supply is therefore an important and inevitable aspect of the regulation of fetal growth. This is an example of maternal constraint (Gluckman and Hanson 2004). An impaired growth trajectory may become irreversible if fetal under-nutrition is prolonged (Mellor and Murray 1982).

This change is clearly of benefit to the fetus, enabling it to optimize the use of limited nutrients, but it may have postnatal costs. If the developing organism increases its chances of survival by, for example, economizing on the building of structures that would have been helpful to it in later life, the short-term gain of survival may be at the expense of its subsequent reproductive success, long-term health, and longevity. In such cases, the risks of failing to survive by devoting too many resources to growth have to be balanced against the risks of failing to reproduce, which is, of course, the goal of all organisms.

This results in altered pancreatic development, and thereby insulin release (Fowden and Hill 2001), and the pathways by which insulin exerts its effects on tissues are changed (Ozanne et al 2003), as well as the growth of blood vessels supplying nutrients to highly metabolically active tissues (Bennis-Taleb et al 1999). All these processes lead to a level of "insulin resistance" that economizes on energy consumption. If the offspring is reared in an energy-poor environment, then such attributes may be advantageous and the individual is more likely to survive to reproduce. Conversely, if the individual is reared in a nutritionally rich postnatal environment, then it may be adversely affected by insulin resistance. This example shows how a prenatal survival strategy may have long-term costs in some environments, causing glucose intolerance, insulin resistance, and obesity with pathological consequences, such as the development of type 2 diabetes.

Timing of Developmental Influences

When does the process of our genes interacting with our environment (our fetal programming) begin? It turns out that evolution has built in the capability to make last-minute, fine-tuning adjustments to our anticipated environment into our genetic toolbox, just like the Australian rabbits and Darwin's finches. We have a critical window or windows to fine-tune the expression of our genes. This is the root of epigenetics, or the science of gene expression as opposed to the study of changes in the genetic code itself.

Our genetic inheritance is technically called our *genotype*. The physical manifestation of our genotype is called our phenotype. So what we are talking about here is *phenotype plasticity*. An organism is always trying to adapt to its environment the best it can, like the rabbits growing bigger ears to cool off in the heat or the finches developing bigger, stronger beaks to eat tougher seeds. Genetic changes, in most cases, require tens of thousands, if not millions, of years. It took approximately 6–7 million years from the time when our line shared a common ancestor with chimpanzees to arrive at anatomically modern humans *(Homo sapiens)*. So our genetics are not going to change from one generation to the next (from your parents to you), but the timeframe for epigenetic changes is much more rapid.

It may surprise you to learn that this process of developmental adjustment actually begins in your grandmother's womb. How can that possibly be? Let's think this through. When your mother was in her mother's womb (your grandmother's womb), the egg that became you was already in your mother before she was born. As you may know, a woman gets all the eggs she will ever have before she is born. Therefore, the genes (half) that will become you were already interacting with an environment: Your grandmother's in utero environment. The point being this: Your grandmother's health, diet, weight and body fat, blood sugar levels, and stress levels—to name only a few environmental factors—impacted your mother's biology and metabolism and also the egg that became you.

Since we can't change our past, what can we do now? If you are contemplating getting pregnant and/or have a child or grandchild who is considering getting pregnant, the time for prospective parents to take the best care of themselves is *before* conception. To create the healthiest baby, you want the healthiest egg and the healthiest sperm possible, because the next crucial window when major changes take place is in the developmental process called conception.

Once the new child is conceived, the maternal environment is crucial. The developing child in the mother's womb makes last-minute decisions about its phenotype based on the environment it predicts it will be born into from the cues of its maternal environment. If the developing child guesses right, the child will be well matched to its environment and thrive. But if it guesses wrong, the child will be mismatched or maladapted to its environment, and it will struggle with metabolic challenges such as excess body fat, blood sugar issues, diabetes, hypertension, and heart disease.

There are a series of critical windows when the newly fertilized egg begins to make these permanent, irreversible "decisions." The first set of decisions takes place at the moment of conception. Another set of decisions takes place when the zygote (the fertilized egg) consists of only four cells. Another set of decisions takes place when the zygote consists of only eight cells. By the third day following conception, the cells have divided to form a small ball known as a blastocyst. By the fourth day, the cells begin to differentiate. By day five, cavitation takes place: the cells of the blastocyst form a fluid-filled cavity with a group of cells clumped at one end of the cavity. On day seven, the blastocyst sinks into the endometrium (the inner wall of the mother's uterus) and implants itself.

During the second week of development after conception, the inner cell mass of the blastocyst structure separates into three distinct layers. The outer layer is known as the ectoderm, which will later form the skin, hair, sweat glands, salivary glands, and the nervous tissue including the brain. The middle layer, or mesoderm, will form muscles, bones, blood, circulatory system, teeth, connective tissues, and kidneys. The inner layer, the endoderm, will form most of the internal organs (stomach, intestines, liver, lungs, and heart).

You can begin to appreciate how vulnerable this newly forming organism is to the maternal environment. And most women still have no idea they are pregnant yet. So, if you are smoking, drinking alcohol, and/or under heavy stress, this will affect the growing organism inside you.

What kind of cues does the developing child get from its mother?

If the mother is undernourished, the developing child will not receive the nutrition it needs to grow and develop optimally. The developing child will make decisions, such as conserving the energy it is getting from the mother via the placenta so it can merely survive. As a result, the developing child's body will be compromised. The child will not only be smaller and born with a low birth weight, but the growth of all of its organs will be compromised. Its heart will be smaller and weaker. Its liver will be smaller and weaker, as well as its kidneys. The child is not just smaller; it will be less able to survive and adapt. Its life will be permanently and irreversibly compromised.

Out of necessity, the fetus chooses a survival phenotype. A survival phenotype is designed to conserve energy, stay alive, get born alive, reproduce as soon as possible, and invest no energy or resources in repair or maintenance of the body. Studies of survivors of the Dutch winter famine of 1944–1945 illustrate the specific long-term consequences of nutrient deprivation during pregnancy (Ravelli et al 1998; Ravelli et al 1999). In November 1944, the Nazi occupiers of Holland imposed severe rationing on the western Netherlands. For seven months, the Dutch, including pregnant women, only received an average of between four hundred and eight hundred calories per day. These pregnant mothers were not only severely malnourished; they were also experiencing high levels of wartime stress. These intense wartime conditions meant these pregnant women had high levels of cortisol, the most powerful stress hormone in the human body. The mothers who were pregnant during this time of imposed famine and major stress gave birth to smaller babies. Underscoring the developmental origins of disease model, these children had much higher levels of obesity, insulin resistance, and heart disease as they got older. The children of women starved during the third trimester experienced the worst health and disease consequences in later life.

The female offspring of women exposed to famine in Holland in 1944/45 in turn gave birth to growth-impaired infants (Lumey 1992). Since changes induced in the fetus may affect metabolic and cardiovascular function when these offspring in turn become pregnant, these outcomes may then induce particular phenotypes in the *next* generation of offspring (Drake and Walker 2004; Gluckman and Hanson 2004), as well.

To exacerbate the problem, this low birth weight child is actually born into a modern world of abundance and excess. The result is often called *catch-up*. The low birth weight child begins to try to catch up to a normal weight. The only problem is that because its metabolism is compromised, most of the weight it gains is fat weight, not muscle weight. The child puts on weight and fat very quickly and often ends up being an overweight or obese child.

What if the mother is diabetic or if she eats a diet high in sugar and/or refined carbohydrates? Then the child developing in her womb will develop what's called metabolic syndrome. Metabolic syndrome is a combination of different metabolic disorders including glucose intolerance and insulin resistance. A person with metabolic syndrome tends to put on fat easily, has high blood sugar levels, is tired all the time, often feels depressed, has high triglyceride levels, and is hungry all the time, among other symptoms.

Bear in mind, the fetus is 100 percent dependent on the oxygen and glucose it must have to stay alive in the womb. If there is a shortage of oxygen because the mother is a smoker, the fetus panics and makes radical adjustments to stay alive long enough to get born alive. If the mother is undernourished (not getting enough calories) or malnourished (the mother is eating a junk food diet), the fetus chooses a survival phenotype. To simply survive during development, the fetus conserves all resources for the most crucial organs—especially the brain—and compromises everything else. The threatened fetus' strategy is to be born alive and reproduce as soon as possible (early puberty), with no concern for maintenance and repair for later life. Remember, the biological point of life is the replication of DNA. So if the fetus perceives a dire environment, its "job" is to stay alive and reproduce to pass along the DNA with the hopes that the environment will improve for future generations.

Once the infant is born, the most important factors are loving care and proper nutrition in infancy and early childhood, as lack of these also has long-term consequences. Loving handling of a baby has long-term consequences on the regulation of cortisol release. Babies deprived of loving care grow up over-reactive to stress, with low serotonin levels and a tendency to depression. Poor nutrition (too little nutrition, nutrition that is deficient in nutrients or junk food, and/or nutrition that is calorically too high) in human babies can have long-term metabolic consequences (Singhal et al 2003), and the resultant impaired infant growth patterns may lead to disease risks in adult life (Eriksson et al 2001).

As a child, I experienced a situation that I now realize perfectly illustrated the power of loving care and nutrition and its impact upon development. When I was about ten years old, my best friend John and I went to the local county fair. One of the games was tossing nickels and trying to get one to stay on a plate. If you succeeded, you won a baby duckling. I was a fat, awkward kid who never won anything. Don't ask me how or why, but for some odd reason I seemed to have a knack for tossing a nickel and getting it to stay on an elevated plate. I won four baby ducklings. Needless to say, I was thrilled. My best friend John didn't win anything. So I gave him two of my baby ducklings.

Over the next six months, I gave my baby ducklings the very best care and food I possibly could. They grew up big and healthy. They were fully grown ducks with beautiful white feathers. The only problem was, they made such a mess on our back patio that my parents said they had to go. So the plan was to take them up to my grandfather's ranch. John's parents, it turned out, felt the same way about his ducks.

So the day arrived to take all four ducks up to my grandfather's ranch. When we drove by to pick up John's ducks, I was shocked. John's ducks were half the size of my ducks, and their feathers had only come half in.

They were half scrawny duck down and half immature white feathers.

So here we have a classic illustration. Obviously, all four ducks were genetically identical. The 4 ducks had been divided into two groups totally randomly. One pair of ducks had been given optimal care and food. The other pair had been neglected and malnourished. The contrast could not have been more stark. I did not realize it at the time, but I had just been given a lesson about the power of optimal nutrition and optimal care.

The moral of this story is simple: While we (or any organism) are developing, we are at our most vulnerable to environmental influences.

The longer-term effects of environmental influences in early life, however, become even more important as longevity becomes a greater feature of the human species. As we've discussed, a functional and evolutionary approach suggests that pregnant women may signal to their unborn babies about their future world. If the fetal forecast is wrong, however, the offspring is at greater health risk because its physiological adaptations are mismatched with the environment in which he or she will live. Gluckman and Hanson (2004) suggested that the fetal environment was likely to match the postnatal environment during most of hunter-gatherer evolution. However, the rapid advances in longevity in recent times, together with the extreme changes in the postnatal nutritional/energy environment have created a greater probability of mismatch (Gluckman and Hanson 2004c).

The rapid growth of a low birth weight baby is one such key risk factor (Barker et al 2002; Eriksson et al 2001). Evidence suggests that the growing baby may be interpreting the abundant availability of nutrition as permissive release from the constraint of fetal life (Gluckman and Hanson 2004; Eriksson et al 1999), which is likely to introduce complexity into the relationship between developmental prediction and later health.

For example, some populations will have adapted to conditions of nutritional stress, especially seasonal food shortages, over a long time span (Truswell and Hansen 1976), while others will have been buffered from such effects. This leads to actual genetic differences, and therefore the existence of actual different genotypes between populations (Hattersley and Tooke 1999; Neel 1999; Diamond 2003). Remember, a genotype is your genetic inheritance. Recent studies (Eriksson et al 2002, 2003) demonstrate that the capacity of early environmental influences to affect later disease risk can be influenced by these genotypes. The possibility of a "thrifty genotype" (Neel 1962), or one that can thrive in a nutritionally scarce environment, may actually be well adapted to harsh conditions and is therefore not incompatible with the "deprivation-adapted phenotype" (fetuses and babies that develop with compromised nutrition). However, should that environment change and become nutrient rich (as in the case of developing countries), it may put such populations at greater risk. Therefore, when studying populations, we must consider environmental factors that act on development, alongside genetic factors, if we are to understand the origins of many human diseases and prevent the existence of generations of "chronically ill, chronically mismatched populations."

Your Developmental Challenge

So what does the developmental challenge have to do with losing weight?

We human beings are like the rabbits in Australia and the finches in the Galapagos Islands. Evolution has programmed us to thrive in a certain environment. Fortunately, we human beings have a huge environmental niche in which we are able to thrive. Think of human beings living and thriving in environments anywhere from the freezing cold Arctic north to hot, steaming equatorial jungles. Think of your genetic inheritance and developmental plasticity as being like a jukebox. As your genes interact with the environment, a tune is chosen that is mostly appropriate for the given environment. The genes don't change, but the expression of the genes do.

As a result, we have a certain degree of plasticity or flexibility as to how our genes will be expressed as we develop (West-Eberhard 2003). The process of developmental plasticity silences or activates certain genes based on the environment we anticipate being born into. These adaptations are called *predictive adaptive responses* (Gluckman, Hanson 2005, 2008).

We have certain critical windows during which permanent irreversible decisions are made. This developmental process begins in your grandmother's womb, intensifies in your mother's womb, and is amplified as you grow up. It continues to this day. If your grandmother or mother were undernourished or had health issues, you were probably affected. If you were born small (less than 5.5 pounds) and then gained weight rapidly (catch-up growth), it permanently affected your metabolism.

All these changes came about because the fetus is reading the cues it is getting from its maternal environment and makes a prediction, kind of like a weatherman. But as we all know, sometimes the weatherman is wrong.

Based on the weatherman's prediction, we might put on shorts, T-shirt, and sandals in anticipation of warm, sunny weather. But when we get to the beach, it might be stormy, windy, and cold. We are ill-prepared for the real environment we find ourselves in.

The consequences of being mismatched with our environment often show up in the form of metabolic disorders. We gain weight more easily than others. We love sugar and carbohydrates, but they don't seem to love us. We may have high blood pressure or diabetes. All of these problems had their origins during our development, especially in our mother's womb. In terms of losing weight (attaining our ideal body weight and sustaining an optimal, healthy weight), it may mean that our road is a little bit steeper than it might otherwise have been. We can still get and stay lean and healthy. We will just have to be a little bit more organized and a little bit more disciplined than maybe some other people. Life is not fair. That is a given. But complaining about it or feeling sorry for yourself will not change a thing. We all have assets and liabilities. What may come easily for us in some areas of our life may be a real challenge to other people, and vice versa. We have to learn to take the good with the bad and to make the best of the hand we were dealt. We will show you exactly how to lose weight, get lean, and achieve optimal health regardless of your developmental challenge.

Chapter 3

The Environmental Challenge

Keep your house clean because…if it's in your house, you (and your family) will eat it.

—Joe Dillon

In previous chapters, we discussed how your genetic and developmental inheritance set the stage for your interactions with the modern environment. In this chapter, we'll explain why even though we live in an obesogenic environment (one that literally encourages obesity and degenerative diseases), not everyone is fat, diabetic, or dies of heart disease.

During our earliest history as hunter-gatherers living on the savanna of East Africa, we lived in an environment we had evolved over millions of years to be suited for. We had long legs and tall, slender bodies with tremendous energy and endurance, and we could walk for miles a day. We had the biggest brains relative to our body size of any organism on earth. We had developed lethal hunting tools and hunting skills. We had gained control of fire and cooked our food. We lived in small bands of 20–30. We were all related to one another. We all cared about each other. We lived in an egalitarian society: share and share alike. We were extraordinarily healthy, and if we escaped infant mortality (which was high) and infection and lived to be fifty, we had a good chance of living to be eighty, ninety, or even one hundred years old (Lindeberg 2010). In this Paleolithic environment, our air and water were pure. There was no pollution. Our stress levels were low, and we lived a relaxed lifestyle with lots of social interaction. We were never alone or depressed.

Between ten thousand and twelve thousand years ago, our human environment began to radically change. This was the beginning of the agricultural revolution. This change in environment from roving bands of hunter-gatherers to a settled agricultural life was not instantaneous. It took thousands of years for human beings to become competent at cultivating cereal grains and domesticating animals. While it was happening, the vast majority of people on earth still lived a hunter-gatherer lifestyle: a physically active life and the ancestral diet.

Yet in some places, human beings began to settle. Newly agricultural human beings built permanent shelters, raised cereal grains and beans, and domesticated animals. Over time, villages formed. Some of these villages became cities. Nutritionally, cereal grains and beans (both high glycemic load carbohydrates) replaced lean meat as the foundation of the new diet. As agricultural humans ate less protein and ate more and more carbohydrates (sugar), over time they grew smaller (shorter) and had less muscle. Living in close proximity with newly domesticated animals, plus the accumulation of both human and animal waste, led to the birth of communicable diseases.

Unlike hunter-gatherers who could simply move, follow migrating game herds, or forage for more plentiful fruit, the newly agricultural humans became dependent on the success of their crops. When there were droughts, crops failed, and the newly agricultural humans experienced famine for the first time in human history. With ever-larger human settlements came power structures, conflict, and stress: the conflict of the powerful and the powerless; the conflict of the haves and the have-nots. Wars between settlements over scarce resources broke out for the first time in human history. The human population, which had been stable for thousands of years and which was easily and sustainably supported by the earth, began to grow rapidly.

As we jump from the dawn of the agricultural revolution to the start of the twentieth century (circa 1900), there were still over two hundred isolated societies around the world living the ancestral hunter-gatherer lifestyle with the same extraordinary health and leanness. In the period before the Industrial Revolution, during the agricultural revolution, most of the rest of the people lived a communal, rural, hand-to-mouth lifestyle. However, there was still a lot of hard physical work involved, and the diet consisted of completely un-processed food. These farmers had a tough life, but they did not suffer any of the diseases of modern humankind. Even for urbanized people living in the big cities, heart disease, cancer, and obesity were rare—but their communal way of living began to create their own set of diseases. The major causes of death were infectious diseases like pneumonia, tuberculosis, and the flu. In fact, the 1918 Spanish flu pandemic killed an estimated twenty-five million people worldwide—more than all the people who were killed in the First World War. It also killed over 675,000 Americans. One of the great triumphs of the twentieth century was the control of infectious diseases.

Which brings us to the twenty-first century. Obesity is now a worldwide epidemic. The top four causes of death are heart disease, cancer, stroke, and lung disease. So what changed in the twentieth century and, especially, the latter half of the twentieth century?

There were some positive changes. The most important was improved sanitation and the development of antibiotics. And there were some nega-tive changes. The cause of these negative changes could not be genetic, for as you have learned, it takes hundreds of thousands to millions of years for genes to change and evolve. Of all the factors we have discussed so far, the factor that has changed the most radically is our environment. Our modern environment directly contributes to the obesity epidemic (Dietary Guidelines for Americans, USDA 2010).

How rapidly things have changed:

- **In the early 1970s**, the prevalence of obesity was 5 percent for chil-dren ages two to five years; 4 percent for children ages six to eleven years; and 6 percent for adolescents ages twelve to nineteen years.

- **In 2007–2008**, the prevalence of obesity reached 10 percent for chil-dren ages two to five years, 20 percent for children ages six to eleven years, and 18 percent for adolescents ages twelve to nineteen years.

- **In the late 1970s**, 15 percent of adults were obese.

- **By 2008**, 34 percent of adults were obese.

- **In the early 1990s**, zero states had an adult obesity prevalence rate of more than 25 percent.

- **In 2008**, thirty-two states had an adult obesity prevalence rate of more than 25 percent (Flegal KM, Carroll MD, et al; Ogden CL,

Flegal KM, et al; Ogden CL, Carroll MD, et al; CDC). Today, these numbers are even higher.

One factor we all have to deal with is what we call the Black Box of Conventional Wisdom. The Black Box of Conventional Wisdom—better known as marketing—is the body of unexamined assumptions most of us base our lives on.

Here's a classic example of what we are up against in our modern obesogenic environment. We are taught to get up in the morning and start our day with a big glass of pure sugar called orange juice—on an empty stomach, no less. This juice encourages our body to get fat, sick, tired, and depressed. Fruit juice raises insulin, which in turn raises our inflammation levels, which encourages the development of obesity, diabetes, and heart disease. This is especially true for those of us who are sugar sensitive (e.g., glucose intolerant, insulin resistant).

All juice is pure sugar or virtually pure sugar. That's a pretty bold statement, but it's incontrovertibly true. If we compare the Nutrition Facts panel of orange juice (with no sugar added), as well as some other popular juices, to a typical cola drink, here is what we find:

Juice = Sugar

Compare the sugar in:
12 ounces of juice (no sugar added) with
12 ounces (one can) of cola

12 Ounces of:	Cola	Orange Juice	Apple Juice	Grape Juice
Total Carbohydrates (grams)	40g	40g	42g	60g
Sugar (teaspoons)	10 tsp.	10 tsp.	10.5 tsp.	15 tsp.
Protein (grams)	0g	2g	0g	<1g
Fat (grams)	0g	<1g	0g	0g
Calories	160	175	165	240

Note that in all cases, almost no calories, or less than two grams, come from protein. In all cases, almost no calories, or less than one gram, come from fat. There are only three macronutrients: proteins, fats, and carbohydrates. Therefore, if none or almost none of the calories come from protein, and none or almost none of the calories come from fat, that only leaves carbohydrate. And if you look at the amount of sugar (carbohydrates) in cola versus orange juice, you will see they have the same amount of sugar (carbohydrates). In some of the juices, the amount of sugar (carbohydrates) is even *higher*. Let's be perfectly clear: The word carbohydrate is the fancy word for sugar.

So you see, both beverages are literally pure sugar. In fact, all juices are virtually pure sugar, including all fruit juices and all vegetable juices—even fresh squeezed. All juices will spike your insulin.

Insulin is the most powerful fat storing hormone in the human body. Insulin also blocks all mobilization of fat. Any time you spike your insulin, you will store fat for the next eight to twelve hours; any time you spike your insulin, your body will *not* be able to burn any fat for the next eight to twelve hours—even if you exercise. Insulin creates a one-way gate into your fat cells.

Think of the sign at car rental agencies announcing, "Do not back up, or it will result in severe tire damage." Fat goes into your fat cells, but none comes out. We drink orange juice because we are taught that orange juice will enhance our health. And we give fruit juice to our children because we love them and care about their health. Notice the next time you see orange juice advertised on TV. The orange juice company does not say that orange juice is pure sugar. Instead, the orange juice advertisers attempt to manipulate you emotionally. The advertisement showing radiantly healthy people drinking orange juice in a beautiful setting, accompanied by the perfect music, tells us that orange juice is full of fresh air and sunshine. The most current advertisements tout orange juice as the best way to handle the stresses of the day. But starting your day with "pure sugar" called orange juice puts you at a tremendous *disadvantage* when it comes to dealing with stress.

An ad for fruit juice brings together powerful entities: huge corporations that spend hundreds of millions of dollars on advertising every year; highly sophisticated advertising companies that are master manipulators; and last but not least, perhaps the most powerful marketing and manipulation tool ever invented—television. Trust me, these entities will do whatever it takes to be profitable, despite the impact it may have on your health. And it is not the corporations' and advertisers' fault. They are just doing what they are supposed to do: make money. Fortunately, we are here to help you decipher these confusing messages so you can make rational choices, based on fact rather than emotional manipulation.

So when and where does our modern environment begin to impact us? We first learn what to eat, how to eat, when to eat, and how much to eat at home. Growing up, I learned a certain way to eat. I assumed that my family and I were eating a healthy diet. I didn't know any better. And nothing I learned on TV or in school contradicted that assumption. I thought I was fat because I was unlucky. I really did not understand that literally stuffing myself until I could not eat another bite with cake and cookies and ice cream was somehow wrong or unhealthy or unusual. It sure did taste good. And there were my mother and father, setting the example by doing the same thing: stuffing themselves at every meal.

I was also taught distracted eating (eating in front of the television). The television was always blasting away as we sat as a family and had our second and third helpings of dessert. As a kid, I used to stay up along with my parents until the TV went off at 1 AM. Johnny Carson would end and the National Anthem would come on. The National Anthem was the signal for all of us to go to bed. I was not only a fat kid, but I was also constantly exhausted and fell asleep in class. In the eighth grade, I got so exhausted and rundown that I got mononucleosis and had to be hospitalized for several weeks. Then I stayed home for a couple of months and finally went back to school. To get better, I was told to take a nap every afternoon after I had a big bowl of ice cream "to build up my strength." By the time I entered high school, I was fatter than I had ever been in my life. That was my home environment.

When we had family gatherings, especially when we visited my uncle and my cousins on my mother's side, food was the central focus. They would literally sit around all day and eat whole loaves of bread slathered with butter. They grew up grossly overweight and diabetic.

At school, we begin to get the institutionalized version. Our children are taught the Food Pyramid, which is now called The Plate (USDA 2011), as the model of healthy eating. Although we will talk much more in depth about this, anyone with any kind of a metabolic disorder will put on weight and fat like crazy if they eat according to the Food Pyramid or even The Plate.

How would you know if you have a metabolic disorder? If you struggle with weight, that is a big red flag. Acne. Tired all the time. Constantly hungry. Depressed. These are all signs of a metabolic disorder, as are glucose intolerance and insulin resistance. The worst possible diet for a person struggling with weight is a high-carbohydrate diet. Why? Carbohydrates raise insulin, and insulin is the most powerful fat storing hormone in the human body.

Look at the Food Pyramid. The base of the pyramid, the foundation of the entire diet, is 6–11 servings of bread, cereal, rice, and pasta. These are all carbohydrates. The next level up is 3–5 servings of vegetables, which although much healthier carbohydrates than bread and pasta, are still carbohydrates. Also on the next level are 2–4 servings of fruit. Unlike fruit juice, whole fruit is healthy, but again, it's another carbohydrate. The next level up includes dairy products. Some people can tolerate dairy products, but many people cannot. Also, dairy products are high in lactose, which is a simple sugar (more carbohydrates). For people who are glucose (sugar) intolerant and/or insulin resistant, all dairy products should be avoided to lose weight.

Also on level three are meat, poultry, fish, dry beans, eggs, and the nuts group. Level three is supposed to be the protein group. But beans are actually one of the highest glycemic load carbohydrates a person can eat and should be avoided by anyone who struggles with weight. And raw nuts, although healthy, are much more of a fat source than a protein source. And, of course, at the peak of the pyramid are fats, oils, and sweets.

The Food Pyramid is really a high-carbohydrate, low-protein, and moderate-fat diet. For those of us (including Sandy and me) who are carbohydrate intolerant, the Food Pyramid is guaranteed to make you fat, tired, and depressed. And this is what is taught in our schools and is the official program of the USDA.

The latest dietary guidelines of The Plate are not much of an improvement (See Table 2-4).

Table 2-4: Recommended Macronutrient Proportions by Age			
	Carbohydrates	Protein	Fat
Young Children (1–3 years)	45-65%	5-20%	30-40%
Older Children (4–18 years)	45-65%	10-30%	25-35%
Adults (19 years and older)	45-65%	10-35%	20-35%

(Source: Institute of Medicine. Dietary Reference Intakes for Energy, Carbohydrate, Fiber, Fat, Fatty Acids, Cholesterol, Protein, and Amino Acids. Washington DC: The National Academies Press 2002).

Here we have in black and white the most current recommendations, as of 2011. We find it interesting that the most current report came out in June 2011, but the recommendations are almost ten years old. We also find it interesting that the most current dietary recommendations state that we should eat half to two-thirds of all of our calories in the form of sugar (carbohydrates). Sandy and I know that if we ate like that, we'd be fat as pigs. We have also experienced the horrible blood panel results we received when we were living on such a diet (remember my story and my elevated cholesterol, among my other issues). Blood tests, which are empirical and don't lie, only further validates how destructive this lifestyle is. And yet these are the official dietary recommendations put out by the United States Department of Agriculture, which is quoting the Institute of Medicine.

What is the average person to think? This is all part of the obesogenic environment, which is actually named in this very report as a cause of the obesity epidemic. How bizarre is that?

At school, not only are our kids taught that the Food Pyramid is healthy (setting them up for a life of obesity and metabolic diseases), but if you take a look at typical school lunches, what chance do our kids have? And we wonder why 20 percent of our children are literally obese.

Now think about holidays and social gatherings. Sugar and binge eating have been institutionalized into our national holidays. Think of Halloween. We teach our children to go out and get grocery bags filled with sugar. Or what would Easter be without big chocolate bunnies or jellybean–filled eggs? Or Thanksgiving, where it is almost unpatriotic not to eat one's self into oblivion and pass out on the couch with a football game blasting away. This is all part of the obesogenic environment. Obesogenic means that our environment literally encourages obesity and the metabolic diseases that go with it.

It's not just holidays. What would a kid's birthday be without pizza and soda and birthday cake or an ice cream cake? A forty-four ounce soda contains 512 calories of pure sugar. What about sporting events like the Super Bowl? At Super Bowl parties, we are surrounded by beer, soda, pizza, and chips and dip as we all passively watch the game.

Cheap, processed junk food is available everywhere. Many convenience stores are open twenty-four hours a day. On top of that, we are inundated with marketing showing us famous lean athletes and attractive celebrities drinking and eating junk food.

In fact, so much of socializing is organized around food and alcohol, it is almost impossible to avoid it. At a restaurant, the first question is, "What would you like to drink?" Alcohol is a popular social lubricant. Alcohol is, of course, the most concentrated of all sugars. Alcohol lowers our inhibitions and stimulates our appetite, so we order more food at the restaurant, and the restaurant makes more money. Alcohol relaxes our smooth muscles so we don't even realize how much food we've eaten or how stuffed we already are.

Then there is the concept of food as a reward. Think of a Happy Meal. As you begin to understand a healthier way of eating for you and your children (if you have them), you will quickly realize there is nothing happy about a Happy Meal. These fast-food meals are just a gimmick to get kids addicted to sugar and grease and to create a future customer.

The next environmental influence contributing to our obesogenic environment is the lack of physical activity. Our ancestors were physically active their entire lives. When I was growing up, an hour of physical education was mandatory from the first grade through senior year in high school. The only students excused from PE class were the athletes on varsity teams who worked out intensely several hours day. By contrast, most schools today have no physical education whatsoever.

Our modern environment encourages a passive, sedentary way of life. We drive everywhere in our cars and park as close as we can. We keep our refrigerator and our cupboards stocked with our favorite snacks so we don't run out. We play video games for hours while snacking on junk food. We order-in pizza and watch the game on our big screen TV at home. Many, if not most of us, work at a sedentary job. At work, we are surrounded by jars of candy, boxes of donuts, and birthday cake. We may even buy lunch off the local "roach-coach" because it is "easy, convenient, and cheap." You can see why it is tough to lose weight and keep it off in our modern environment.

In addition, studies have shown that fat is contagious (Christakis 2007). Research shows that people are more likely to become obese when a friend becomes obese. If a friend became obese, that increased a person's chances of becoming obese by 57 percent. The greatest influence of all was between mutual close friends. With mutual close friends, if one became obese, the odds of the other becoming obese nearly tripled.

Our modern environmental challenge has multiple aspects. The first and most glaring is a diet high in sugar, refined carbohydrates, and unhealthy fat. The food is calorically dense, but low in nutrients. It is easy to take in a lot of calories without realizing it. At the same time, these calories give you no nutritional benefit, causing us to become overweight but malnourished. And if we try to make healthy changes in our eating habits, oftentimes it is our family and our best friends who give us the most grief. All these factors create a kind of inertia. We are pulled passively down. The Black Box of Conventional Wisdom has a powerful gravitational pull.

If we want to lose weight and keep it off in our modern environment, we have to fight against the current. We have to go against the grain (literally and metaphorically). Again, we are not trying to be discouraging. We want you to know we get it. We understand how difficult it is to make healthy choices, and we are on your side.

One thing hopefully may be becoming clear by now. There is only one person in our modern environment who actually cares about your health and the health of your children. *You.* If you don't care, no one cares. So what can you do if you want to lose weight and keep it off?

We evolved over literally millions of years to thrive in a very different environment from today's obesogenic environment. As a result, there is a huge mismatch between how we evolved to live and eat versus the high sugar, high fat, high refined carbohydrate diet we now eat, combined with a passive, sedentary lifestyle.

You need to grasp that the modern environment is not going to be any help. Our environment is full of misinformation and companies selling foods that pander to our worst impulses. Here is a realistic place to start: Accept that our modern environment is a nonstop, twenty-four-hour-a-day obesogenic challenge. You can succeed, but you have to be prepared and get organized. Before you get too depressed, it's not like you can never have any fun—we'll show you how to do that as well. But it is important to realize that actions have consequences. For us. For our children.

On the other hand, once you know what you are doing, it is possible to become healthier and leaner than you have ever been before. Sandy and I are living proof of this. You can begin to swing your metabolic pendulum from the weight-gain direction to the weight-loss direction. The more you practice The Joe Dillon Difference lifestyle, the more momentum you will gather. We will teach you how to take control of your environment, starting with your home. We will teach you how to thrive even in our modern environment. Let us show you how.

Chapter 4

The Aging Challenge

Half the world is aging themselves faster by eating lousy diets.

—Bruce Ames, PhD, Professor of Biochemistry
and Molecular Biology at the University of California,
Berkeley, international authority on aging, and author
of over five hundred studies on aging

What does aging have to do with losing weight?

One of the implicit questions of this book and of our research since 1979 is, "What is the optimal biological lifestyle?" How do we live and behave (e.g., eat, exercise, sleep) so we have the highest quality of life (from a biological point of view as opposed to the superficial point of view promoted by mass media) and the maximum quantity of life (live as long as possible)?

As we begin to address the Aging Challenge, once again we must revisit our past. As we look back in evolutionary time, we notice a simple, clear, unchanging biological reality: Every organism gets older. We human beings evolved over 6–7 million years to become anatomically modern humans approximately two hundred thousand years ago, and in fact, we humans have one of the longer lifespans. But, the reality is, we humans get older too. So, given the fact that we all age, it makes sense to us to do everything known to science to slow down or delay the biological process of aging and do everything known to science to avoid accelerating the biological process of aging.

As we get older, our body changes. That is just the reality of aging. Our body becomes less resilient. As we age, it takes our body longer to recover from setbacks. Notice the difference in response between your body and that of a young child. If a young child gets a nick or a cut, all evidence of that injury is completely gone in just a few days. This remarkable healing power holds true from birth up until about age thirty (the end of our peak reproductive years). After about age thirty, the aging process really begins to kick in. Why? Recall that from a strictly biological perspective, the point of life is to pass on our DNA to the next generation. During this window (from birth to the end of our peak reproductive years), our body's repair mechanisms are nearly perfect. Once we pass our prime reproductive years, our body puts very little energy or resources into maintenance and repair. Our body has served its biological purpose.

This is true of most animals. One of the most dramatic examples of this total investment in reproduction and zero investment in the post-reproductive body are salmon. After living in the ocean for a number of years, they expend heroic amounts of energy to swim upstream, even jumping waterfalls, to return to where they were born in order to spawn. Once the salmon reach the spawning grounds, they spawn and die within two weeks. The salmon have fulfilled their biological reproductive function. As far as Nature is concerned, the salmon are no longer needed. If we want to slow or delay the aging process, we have to consciously and deliberately compensate for the lack of Nature's help.

So, yes, as we get older, biological mechanisms will also slow down. But that doesn't mean there is nothing we can do about it. Remember, we have a biological age and a chronological age. What does this mean? It means that, although we are all getting older chronologically, there are certain things we can do to create an environment in which our body is functioning as if it were actually younger (e.g., reduce our biological age). Our biological age is made up of a complex of physiological markers. When it comes to losing weight more effectively and efficiently, having a younger biological age is helpful.

Here are some physiological markers that help give you an estimate of your biological age: body fat percentage; waist circumference; strength; resting heart rate; fasting glucose; hemoglobin A1c; triglycerides; fasting insulin; HDL cholesterol; bone density; thyroid status; hormone status (menopause, andropause); sodium/potassium ratio; and resting metabolic rate. Better yet, these are physiological markers of health and aging that you have complete control over.

By addressing the key markers that determine your current biological state, you will learn how to accurately ascertain your current status. Then we will teach you what to do to improve that status, so you not only lose weight, but you lose weight in such a way that you age more successfully.

By giving The Joe Dillon Difference lifestyle a reasonable effort, you will be able to manage and optimize the most important physiological markers of aging. You will be able to safely and effectively lose weight and lower your body fat percentage. You will be able to achieve and sustain your biologically optimal body weight. You will be able to decrease your waist circumference and have a flatter stomach. You will get stronger. Your heart will get stronger; you will get into excellent cardiovascular aerobic shape; and, therefore, you will have a lower resting heart rate. Your fasting glucose will drop well below 100 and into the optimal range (70–85). Your hemoglobin A1c will become optimal.

Hemoglobin A1c is like a running average of your glucose levels and gives you a good picture of how consistently stable you are keeping your blood sugar. Hemoglobin A1c is also an inflammation marker. You will be able to dramatically decrease your triglycerides to well below 100. Lower is better. Your fasting insulin will decrease to the optimal range (6–27 ulU/mL). With the full-body aerobic exercise program we will teach you, you will be able to increase your HDL cholesterol (your good cholesterol) to more than 55 mg/dl (higher is better). You will be able to increase your bone density and have optimal bone health. By checking your thyroid status via blood tests we will recommend, you will able to ascertain the current biological reality of your thyroid and learn if you need thyroid supplementation to regain optimal thyroid functionality. We will also recommend a full inflammation marker panel. You will also be able to optimize your sodium/potassium ratio by cutting back on salt (sodium chloride) and increasing your potassium intake by eating more green vegetables.

And you will be able to ascertain your full hormone status via blood tests we will recommend. We will advise you on the most effective steps to take to optimize your hormone levels. This applies to women with PMS issues, as well as women dealing with menopause. In general, women go through menopause around age fifty, plus or minus a few years. However, men may be surprised to learn that a full hormone panel may be even more important for them. Why? Men begin to go through a major hormonal change, called andropause, at a much younger age. Men actually begin andropause at around age thirty. The root of the word "andropause" is androgen. Androgen is the word for the male hormones, including free testosterone. At approximately age thirty, men's free testosterone begins to decline. It declines slowly at first, and then more rapidly.

As men's free testosterone levels decline, their libido declines. But free testosterone also affects many aspects of men's lives, including their physiological and emotional factors. The optimal free testosterone level for men is 25–35. Many men in their late thirties have single-digit (7, 8 or 9) free testosterone. Their free testosterone is already in the toilet. The two organs in the human body that have the greatest number of receptor sites for free testosterone are your brain and your heart. That means as a man ages and his free testosterone declines, it is going to be impossible for this man to have a healthy, fully functioning brain and a strong, healthy, fully functioning heart. As men slide deeper into andropause, they lose muscle mass; they get weaker; they put on fat more easily, especially abdominal fat, which is a major health risk; they have less energy; they feel tired all the time; they have trouble sleeping; emotionally, they get grumpy, irritable, or angry. They may fly into a rage. By the time men get into their fifties and sixties, andropause is a major cause of depression and suicide.

In addition to measuring free testosterone, men should also learn what their estradiol level is. Estradiol is a form of estrogen. As men slide deeper into andropause, their body produces more aromatase. Aromatase is an enzyme that converts the man's already declining levels of free testosterone into estrogen. It is not uncommon for married men in their fifties to be producing more estrogen than their wives. One symptom of elevated levels of estrogen is the presence of "man breasts" (gynecomastia). Estrogen also makes men fat, and in turn, excess body fat produces even more estrogen. So an overweight man in andropause can get caught in a vicious cycle.

We can teach you how to break out of this cycle and also how to minimize your andropause. The place to start is to get a full hormone panel (see the Resources at the back of this book). We will, of course, also address optimal hormone levels for women.

Another reality of aging is that we can't burn calories or fat as fast at sixty as we did at eighteen years of age. If we overeat at a given meal, it takes much longer for that meal to clear. Not only does our metabolism slow down, it changes. You learned about the impact of development on metabolism. If we discover we have metabolic disorders (we gain weight easily, are glucose intolerant, insulin resistant, and/or diabetic), these metabolic issues will only become more challenging as we get older.

However, growing older does not mean you are defeated. Growing older simply means the dynamic balance becomes more precarious. You can't get away with indiscretions the way you used to. You pay a bigger price for eating too much, eating the wrong thing, drinking too much, or not getting enough sleep. If your metabolic pendulum gets going in the wrong direction (you gain weight), it takes longer and more work to stop the negative direction, and longer still to get your metabolic pendulum to swing back in a positive direction (the place where you start losing weight again). Even Sandy and I deal with that reality. Being lean at eighteen is one thing. Being lean at thirty is another. Being lean at fifty is a bigger challenge and much more of an accomplishment. Someone once said, "You have the face you were born with at eighteen; you have the face you earned at fifty."

Not only will The Joe Dillon Difference teach you how to lose weight, we will also teach you how to enhance your metabolism. You will learn how to attain and sustain optimal health and full functionality for as long as possible. An optimal biological lifestyle increases not only your life span but, more importantly, your health span—because as you age, you not only want a "long" life, but you want to avoid the "disability zone." This is a very important aspect of aging. So much of aging is simply neglect.

Many people have never exercised in their lives, so as they get older, it catches up with them. They are weak and out of shape. If not properly stimulated, your body and your metabolism will fail. Use it or lose it. Many older people are so weak they can't even climb a single flight of stairs or stand up on their own. One of the things Sandy and I enjoy is going to the theater. Our favorite Sunday date is dinner and a play. We are always amazed at how slow many of the people walk at these plays. They move like frail ninety-year-olds, and many may even need a walker or a wheelchair. Yet many of them are younger than Sandy and me. Also, I fly one hundred thousand to two hundred thousand miles a year. Over the years, I have noticed a changing pattern. When I first began to travel intensely, I only rarely saw a person wheeled onto a plane in a wheelchair. Now it is not uncommon to see eight or ten people lined up in wheelchairs, all waiting to be pushed onboard the plane, some with oxygen bottles. And most of these people in wheelchairs are younger than I am! The Joe Dillon Difference lifestyle will teach you how to avoid the "disability zone."

You need to stimulate your body if you want to lower your biological age and avoid becoming one of those people I have just discussed. Proper exercise not only improves your muscle strength, but it bestows many more positive benefits. There is a measure of work in exercise physiology called a met. A met is one metabolic rate, or the number of calories your body burns at rest. As you begin to exercise, you work at a higher and higher met level. So for example, if you are working at even a moderate level of 5 mets, your metabolism is literally running five times faster than it runs at rest. As you get in better shape, you may be able to work at 8 or even 10 mets. This really stimulates your metabolism.

In addition, it will take your body several hours to calm back down to your resting 1 met level. During this post-exercise time, your metabolism is elevated, and you are burning more calories and more fat. If you exercise regularly, and particularly if you do the kind of full-body aerobic exercise we recommend, it will crank up your metabolism for 8–12 hours after your work out. This is a residual benefit of full-body aerobic exercise. Your furnace will burn hotter, and you will generate more heat after exercise from the food you eat. You will be increasing the thermogenic effect of food. Another major benefit of full-body aerobic exercise is the production of mitochondria. Inside every cell in your body, you have organelles or sub-cells called mitochondria. You have about five hundred mitochondria in every cell. Mitochondria are the little structures inside your cells that convert the food you eat (proteins, fats, and carbohydrates) into energy. One of the benefits of exercise is that it stimulates the production of more mitochondria inside your muscle cells. The more mitochondria you have, the faster your metabolism, and therefore, the more calories and the more fat your body burns twenty-four hours a day. By doing full-body aerobic exercise, you are stimulating over 90 percent of your lean body mass to produce more mitochondria.

As it turns out, mitochondria are a major component in the aging equation. Bruce Ames, PhD, is a professor of biochemistry and molecular biology at the University of California, Berkeley. Dr. Ames is one of the world's foremost authorities on the aging process, and he has published over five hundred peer-reviewed scientific articles on aging. Dr. Ames has been studying the molecular biology of mitochondria and their relationship to aging since his doctoral studies in the 1950s at the California Institute of Technology. Dr. Ames and his lab have discovered that mitochondrial decay is involved in all the degenerative diseases of aging, including cancer, heart disease, and brain dysfunctions such as Alzheimer's. He has also discovered that two supplements can renew mitochondria and therefore delay the aging process. We will talk about both of these supplements in the Supplementation chapter later in this book. To us, it makes sense to avoid anything that accelerates mitochondrial decay (such as lack of aerobic exercise) and do everything you can to enhance the number and quality of the mitochondria in your body.

Dr. Ames has also discovered how vitamin and mineral (micronutrient) deficiencies accelerate the aging process and how common micronutrient deficiencies are. One of the ironies of the obesity epidemic is that people are both overfed and undernourished. One of the things that drives hunger are micronutrient deficiencies. If you are low on a critical micronutrient, like magnesium for example, you will stay hungry and keep eating in an effort to satisfy that micronutrient need. In the Supplementation chapter later in this book, we will share some of the specific micronutrient deficiencies that Dr. Ames has discovered, and exactly what to do to correct them. If you want to delay the aging process, it makes sense to avoid anything that depletes your body of essential micronutrients. Some of these deleterious substances are sugar, high fructose corn syrup, refined carbohydrates, and alcohol. So, instead, shouldn't you do everything you can to optimize micronutrient levels in your body, instead of destroying them?

The next important concept to remember when trying to lower your biological age is that you age from your brain down. We are very plastic early in development. But over time, we become less plastic. The one organ, however, that remains plastic throughout your entire life is your brain. So part of The Joe Dillon Difference lifestyle is learning how to take extraordinarily good care of your brain. Like most other things in life, your brain is also, an example of "use it or lose it." Aerobic exercise is the single best thing you can do to keep your brain young and functional. It also turns out that one of the best things you can do for your brain is to stay as lean as possible and to keep a flat stomach. Last but not least, being mentally active, as opposed to passive, is another important activity for brain health. For example, watching TV (a passive activity) does nothing to stimulate brain growth and plasticity, but reading a good book (an active activity) does.

On the other hand, despite what the Black Box of Conventional Wisdom (marketing) teaches us, drinking alcohol is one of the worst things you can do for your brain. All alcohol, including red wine, is neurotoxic. Neurotoxic means that even a four-ounce glass of red wine kills brain cells by the thousands. Not only does alcohol destroy your brain cells, but the damage does not stop there. According to the most comprehensive study on cancer done in human history, which was first released in November 2007, alcohol use is extremely detrimental if you want to avoid cancer. A panel composed of dozens of international scientists, including Nobel Prize Laureates, reviewed over seven thousand studies on cancer over a five-year period. This international panel of scientists made eight unanimous recommendations, including minimizing your intake of alcohol (Diet and Nutrition Cancer Report 2007).

Alcohol is yet another example of marketing versus biological facts. If you look at alcohol through the lens of evolutionary biology, you will realize that our pre-agricultural ancestors drank zero alcohol. Our pre-agricultural ancestors had no dementia, no senility, and no Alzheimer's. We have come to accept these cognitive dysfunctions as an inevitable part of the aging process, but they are not inevitable. Remember, there is no cure for these problems. The only effective approach to cognitive dysfunctions is prevention.

So once again we find ourselves looking at our body through the lens of evolutionary biology and the influences of environment. It is important to remain aware of the impact of your evolutionary past, as well as the impact of your development and the impact of your environment.

We often speak about the Black Box of Conventional Wisdom. People talk about *thinking* outside the Box of Conventional Wisdom. We are advocating that you *live* outside the Box of Conventional Wisdom. For example, conventional wisdom teaches us that as we get older, we get fatter. We are mistakenly led to believe that putting on excess body fat is just a natural part of the aging process. In fact, putting on excess body fat as we age is not natural. Getting fat as we age is only a "natural" part of the process of getting older for people who are living an urbanized, modern sedentary life and eating simple sugars, high fructose corn syrup, refined carbohydrates, processed cereals, refined flour products, high-fat meats, processed meats, processed oils, and salty foods. Traditional peoples living a hunter-gatherer lifestyle did not get fat as they got older. They stayed lean and fit throughout their long and healthy lives.

Conventional wisdom tells us that as we get older, our blood pressure will "naturally" go up; that we will get weaker; that we can't build muscle or get stronger; that we don't need as much sleep; that our posture will "naturally" fail and we will be stooped over; that it is only "natural" that we will need to take more and more drugs; and that we will "naturally" become sicker and sicker.

In the late 1980s and early 1990s, Dr. Staffan Lindeberg, MD, PhD, did an extensive research project on the Kitavans, one of the last remaining isolated peoples living a pre-agricultural, hunter-gatherer lifestyle. In his book, he showed pictures of Kitavans who were over ninety years old. These old Kitavans were lean, fit, and robustly healthy. Dr. Lindeberg reported that he found no cognitive problems: no senility, dementia, or Alzheimer's. All the Kitavans, young and very old, had clear minds and sharp memories (Lindeberg 2010). Studies on over 229 different cultures of traditional peoples worldwide living an ancestral lifestyle proved that their blood pressure did not go up. In fact, as they got older, their blood pressure actually went down. As these traditional peoples grew older, they maintained good strength levels and strong bones. They stood erect with good posture. They had no trouble sleeping seven to nine hours a night. They took no drugs and had none of the degenerative diseases that currently plague modern, urbanized human beings.

So much of life is a self-fulfilling prophecy. It is important not to get caught in the Black Box of myth, ignorance, and misperception. One of the best lessons in life is to pick good role models. If you want to age successfully, naturally, and biologically, versus all the superficial, fake, and cosmetic aging of plastic surgery and Botox we see so much of in the media today, find some healthy role models. Our environment gives us false and misleading information about growing old and the aging process.

That being said, yes, as we grow older, losing weight becomes more of a challenge. But just like the challenges we have already discussed, the challenge of aging can also be overcome.

Start With a Baseline

One of the keys to losing weight is to start by assessing your biological baseline with a comprehensive blood panel and an accurate body composition test. As you begin to practice The Joe Dillon Difference lifestyle, you will keep track of your results. By practicing, measuring, and recording, you will discover your own areas of vulnerability and susceptibility, as well as your thresholds in each of these areas. For example, you will quickly discover if you are metabolically challenged by carbohydrates and what your carbohydrate threshold is, meaning how much carbohydrate can you tolerate before your blood sugar spikes. Stable blood sugar is essential to losing weight, controlling inflammation, and delaying the aging process. Again, The Joe Dillon Difference is about getting in touch with the biological reality of *your* body and then learning how to behave (e.g., eat, drink, sleep, exercise, supplement) in such a way that you optimize your body fat percentage, your energy, and your health. If you know what you are doing (and we will teach you exactly what to do, how to do it, and how to empirically measure your results), you can lose weight and maintain a much younger biological age. With a biological age younger than your chronological age, you will look better, feel better, and be optimally healthy. And it will be real. Not some phony façade. If you are anything like Sandy and me, once you get fully engaged in this process, you will find it fascinating and rewarding. One of our goals for you is that you be disease-free and drug-free for the rest of your long and healthy life.

Chapter 5

The Inflammation Challenge

Inflammation: The Silent Killer
—*Time* Magazine Cover Story, 2004

The Inflammation Challenge is an important aspect of this book. It is now scientific consensus that chronic inflammation is the root cause of virtually all degenerative diseases, including heart disease, cancer, stroke and Alzheimer's.

That's the bad news. The good news is that each of us has virtually 100 percent control over the level of inflammation in our body. Weight loss or, more accurately, fat loss is directly relevant to inflammation because excess body fat is one of the major causes of chronic inflammation. So here we have yet another compelling reason to get leaner. Your body fat percent is a good indicator of the level of systemic inflammation in your body. As we have said so often: Leaner is better. Leaner is healthier. As you learn to lose the right kind of weight (fat weight), you will be simultaneously reducing your inflammation levels and reducing your risk of degenerative disease.

Aging is a complex, multifactorial process, and inflammation is an equally dynamic, complex, and multifactorial process. To understand inflammation, you first need to establish your inflammation baseline with a series of blood tests. Blood tests measure the presence and amounts of specific biologic molecules in your blood, including inflammation markers. To reduce the level of inflammation in your body, you simply have to be willing to make the necessary lifestyle and behavioral changes to eliminate self-inflicted causes of chronic inflammation.

What is inflammation? Fundamentally, acute inflammation is the immune response of tissues due to injury. Clinical characteristics of acute inflammation include pain, heat, swelling, and redness at the site of the injury. This type of acute inflammation is normally a localized, protective response following trauma or infection. Acute inflammation is a normal process that protects and heals the body following physical injury or infection. Acute inflammation is a positive biological mechanism and has been genetically conserved by evolution. Inflammation is another one of those biological two-edged swords. It cuts both ways. Acute inflammation is the positive side. But if inflammation persists and becomes chronic, then it has negative biological effects such as hypertension, heart disease, or Alzheimer's disease.

What are some symptoms of chronic inflammation? If you or your family experiences any kind of respiratory problems such as asthma, allergies, bronchitis, sinusitis, or hay fever, these are all indications of chronic inflammation. You don't need drugs to reduce these symptoms. You simply need to change your diet. And we will teach you exactly how. If you or your family experiences digestive issues such as acid reflux, ulcers, colitis, ileitis, Crohn's disease, or irritable bowel syndrome, these are all symptoms of chronic inflammation. Again, you don't need drugs. You definitely don't need surgery. You simply need to change your diet.

In fact, if you or your family suffer from any problem that ends in "itis," such as bronchitis, arthritis, tendonitis, prostatitis, or gingivitis (gum disease), these are all symptoms of chronic inflammation. For instance, if your gums bleed when you brush and/or floss your teeth, this is a classic symptom of chronic, systemic inflammation. Your dentist can take one look inside your mouth and tell instantly if you have chronic inflammation by the condition of your gums. Your body does not lie. Again, the answer is to change your diet and lifestyle. We want to avoid taking drugs of any kind if we can and for as long as we can. For instance, one of the most commonly used drugs to deal with the pain of chronic inflammation is cortisone. Cortisone and related drugs provide some temporary relief, but in the long run, they actually make the problem worse. For one thing, cortisone type drugs waste away lean body mass and cause fat gain. Loss of lean body mass (muscle) compromises your immune system in major ways. And excess body fat is a major cause of chronic inflammation. Again, you can see the mismatch between the Black Box of Conventional Wisdom (Western medicine and the overemphasis on prescription drugs) and what is congruent with our biological reality.

Where did inflammation come from? When evolution finds something that works, it tends to keep or conserve it. The inflammation response has been conserved for millions of years in our human ancestors. For millions of years, the acute inflammation response helped our ancestors deal with injury and infection. For millions of years, there wasn't much chronic inflammation. Our ancestors either got better or they died. There was not much middle ground, and there were virtually no causes of chronic inflammation.

When did all that change? Somewhere between ten thousand and twelve thousand years ago, the agricultural revolution began. With the agricultural revolution came the cultivation of cereal grains. With the cultivation of cereal grains came a fundamental shift in the human diet. With the agricultural revolution, the foundation of the human diet switched from meat (a high-protein, moderate-fat, low-carbohydrate diet) to cereal grains (a high-carbohydrate, lower-fat, low-protein diet). These changes were gradual at first. As recently as 1900, chronic inflammation was not a major problem. The biggest problems were communicable diseases.

The occurrence of chronic inflammation and its resultant diseases began to show up with the Industrial Revolution. But chronic inflammation and the resultant diseases, such as heart disease and cancer, really took off following the Second World War when the corporate mass-production of processed foods exploded. Following World War II, sugar and refined carbohydrates became cheap. Trans fats (hydrogenated vegetable oil) began to show up in virtually all processed foods. High fructose corn syrup was invented in 1957. The industrial food production process was developed between 1965 and 1970. Since 1975, aided by $40 billion a year in federal subsidies to corn growers, the use of high fructose corn syrup in the United States skyrocketed. Highly processed foods like hydrogenated vegetable oils and high fructose corn syrup are a huge mismatch with our genetic make-up, which developed over millions of years to thrive on lean meat and unprocessed, low glycemic load carbohydrates, such as green leafy vegetables. In the last thirty years, the occurrence of obesity and diabetes has exploded world-wide to epidemic proportions.

Some of us are much more susceptible to biologic insults, such as chronic inflammation, than others. If your mother ate a high-carbohydrate diet and had high levels of insulin during the time you spent in the womb, your body was inflamed in the womb and you are going to be much more susceptible to chronic inflammation. Chronically elevated levels of insulin are one of the major causes of chronic inflammation. If your mother was stressed out and carried high levels of cortisol in her blood (and therefore yours) you will tend to over-react to stress and release more cortisol. Cortisol is the most powerful stress hormone secreted by your body and is one of the major causes of chronic inflammation.

We live in an obesogenic environment. One of your challenges is to find something reasonably healthy to eat in an environment full of simple sugars like candy; highly refined carbohydrates like muffins, breads, and cereals; high fructose corn syrup in drinks like forty-four-ounce soft drinks; and alcohol. All of the things I just mentioned are major contributors to chronic inflammation.

Aging contributes to chronic inflammation because as you get older, your levels of free testosterone and growth hormone decline, along with your lean body mass. At the same time, your levels of insulin and cortisol tend to rise. Elevated insulin, insulin resistance, and glucose intolerance all contribute to chronic inflammation. As many people grow older, they grow weaker and more frail, and, consequently, they become less physically active. A sedentary lifestyle is a major contributor to chronic inflammation.

An increase in your body fat levels and/or a decrease in your lean body mass (muscle) contribute to chronic inflammation. Leaner is better. Less body fat means lower levels of systemic inflammation.

Causes of Chronic Inflammation

What causes chronic, systemic inflammation?

One major cause of chronic inflammation is excess body fat. What do we mean by excess body fat? Excess body fat for men is any body fat over 15 percent. Excess body fat for women is any body fat over 22 percent. Given that the national average for men is 26 percent body fat and for women 36 percent body fat, you can see most people are in trouble. How does excess body fat cause chronic inflammation? People used to think that fat was a passive tissue. But recent research has discovered that fat (or adipose tissue) is actually an endocrine organ. If adipose tissue is an endocrine organ, that means adipose tissue must secrete hormones and hormone-like substances.

In fact, adipose tissue secretes a number of different hormone-like substances. One group of hormones secreted by your fat cells is called pro-inflammatory cytokines. Cytokines are small organic messenger molecules that are dispersed throughout your entire body. Pro-inflammatory cytokines released by adipose tissue amplify inflammatory reactions. Think of pro-inflammatory cytokines as gasoline poured on a fire. The more excess body fat you have, the bigger the adipose endocrine organ and the more pro-inflammatory cytokines your body is secreting twenty-four hours a day. You can begin to see why an overweight person is at a much higher risk for all degenerative diseases: heart disease, cancer, stroke, Alzheimer's, etc. The more fat you have, the higher the level of chronic inflammation throughout your entire body. Less fat, less inflammation. Leaner is healthier.

A second major cause of chronic inflammation is an elevated level of the stress hormone cortisol. Cortisol is the most powerful stress hormone secreted by your body. Anything that raises your cortisol levels will increase your levels of chronic inflammation. What raises cortisol? As one example, a lack of an optimal amount of sleep is stressful and raises cortisol. Optimal sleep is at least seven hours a night, with seven to nine hours a night being a healthy range, regardless of your age. People who try to run on four or five hours of sleep a night are chronically exhausted and are asking for trouble. Also, lack of sleep makes us fat. So now we are compounding our causes of chronic inflammation, with both cortisol and excess body fat. Cortisol is another double-edged biologic sword. We need some cortisol to function and be healthy. But too much cortisol leads to problems. Overtraining is another example of a behavior that raises cortisol. Exercise makes us healthier, but too much exercise or exercise that is too intense will raise our cortisol levels too high. Overtraining will make us fatter. Overtraining depresses our immune system so we are more vulnerable to catching a cold or getting sick. And overtraining that leads to excess cortisol wastes away your lean body mass.

A third major cause of inflammation is excess arachidonic acid. Arachidonic acid is yet another two-edged biological sword. Arachidonic acid is also known as omega-6 fat. Omega-6 and omega-3 fatty acids are the two essential fats. Our body has to have them. Unfortunately, too much of a good thing leads to trouble. The ideal ratio of essential fat intake is 1:1. That means our intake of omega-3 and omega-6 should be equal. In our obesogenic environment, however, the typical ratio is 20:1 omega-6 to omega-3. Excess omega-6 gets converted to a pro-inflammatory prostaglandin called PGE2. These pro-inflammatory molecules feed the fire of inflammation. You have probably heard that trans fats are not healthy. You heard right. One of the reasons trans fats, or partially hydrogenated vegetable oils, are unhealthy is they get converted to excess arachidonic acid. The same thing happens with all the fried foods served at fast-food restaurants. They are dripping with excess pro-inflammatory arachidonic acid that increases inflammation and sets our body up for degenerative disease. There is nothing happy about a Happy Meal.

A fourth major cause of inflammation is excess insulin. Insulin is a hormone secreted by your pancreas. It is a crucial hormone, and you cannot live without it. But, as usual, too much of a good thing leads to trouble. Excess insulin raises your inflammation levels. Insulin is also the *most* powerful fat-storing hormone in your body. So anything that raises insulin will both increase your inflammation levels and make you fatter. What raises insulin? Sugar in all its forms: cakes, pies, ice cream, candy bars, soft drinks, donuts; *all* flour products are pure sugar, including all breads (white and so-called whole grain), breakfast cereals (sweetened and not sweetened), bagels, pancakes, waffles, pasta (white flour pasta and so-called whole wheat pasta), chips, tortillas; any time you overcarb (most of us can only handle up to about twenty-five grams of carbs in a given meal—that's equivalent to about one medium sized apple), or any time you eat carbs of any kind on an empty stomach; and last but not least, all forms of alcohol.

Alcohol, of course, is the most refined of all sugars. To make alcohol, you distill sugar. Alcohol is metabolized by your liver, which turns alcohol into triglycerides. Nothing will raise your triglycerides higher or faster than alcohol. You will learn what the optimal levels of triglycerides are. Suffice it to say: the lower your triglycerides, the better. Alcohol will make you fat (triglycerides get stored directly into your fat cells), and excess body fat raises inflammation levels. Again, you are compounding the inflammation problem: sugar/insulin + excess body fat.

Get Your Comprehensive Blood Panel

I have been working with clients one-on-one since 1979. I have always included comprehensive blood testing as part of my program for all of my clients. I have my clients get a comprehensive blood panel when we first start working together to establish their baselines. Then we retest at the end of the program as proof that the program really did make them healthier. You can't argue with black-and-white blood results. As a result, I have seen literally thousands of blood panels over the last thirty-plus years.

We encourage you to get a comprehensive blood panel if you really want to take charge of your health. Included in a comprehensive blood panel will be a full inflammation marker panel comprising all the major inflammation markers. In the chapter called "Listen to YOUR Body," we will teach you exactly what you should include in your blood panel. We will also teach you what the optimal ranges are for each of your blood values. The blood testing company should send the blood results directly to you, so you can compare your actual results with the ranges for optimal health. Just as one of our goals for you is the optimization of your body composition, we also want you to optimize your blood panel. That way you will know The Joe Dillon Difference really works for you.

What can you do to optimize your inflammation levels?

One of the most effective actions you can take to lower or optimize your inflammation levels is to get and keep your blood sugar levels as stable as possible. You want to avoid triggering an insulin spike, as insulin is a major cause of elevated inflammation levels and your body's most powerful fat storage hormone. The single most effective thing you can do to keep your blood sugar stable is to control the food you eat. The cornerstone of every single meal should be a fist of lean, complete protein (turkey, chicken, fish, egg whites, whey protein isolate shakes) combined with no more than a fist (about a cup) of low glycemic load (slow-burning) carbohydrates (green vegetables being your very best carb). We will teach you how to dial in your lean-protein-to-slow-burning-carb ratio so you lose body fat and have the lowest possible inflammation levels. As a simple rule of thumb: Always remember to eat your lean, complete protein first.

Another effective action you can take to lower or optimize your inflammation levels is to make sure you are getting sufficient amounts of the essential fat omega-3, which is a very powerful anti-inflammatory. The cleanest, purest source of omega-3 is molecularly distilled fish oil. We recommend that you take one to two capsules of molecularly distilled fish oil with each one of your meals, or six to twelve capsules per day.

Optimally healthy meal

Fist of lean protein +
Fist of slow-burning carbs +
Thumb of essential fat or *1–2 caps* of
Super Omega-3

How will you know whether you need six or twelve capsules per day? In the chapter "Listen to YOUR Body," we will help interpret your blood test results, including your inflammation markers, and teach you exactly how to determine what the precise dosage is for *your* optimal health. Your body does not lie. If your inflammation markers are high, a good rule of thumb is that you will probably need the maximum dosage of twelve capsules per day. There is a direct link for Super Omega-3 capsules available on our website.

A major cause of stress, and therefore increased inflammation levels, is elevated cortisol levels, which are exacerbated by chronic lack of sleep. An optimal amount of sound sleep is so important to getting lean and healthy that we will devote an entire chapter to sleep. In the meantime, your goal is to average seven to nine hours of sleep every twenty-four hours (naps count).

Excess body fat is a major contributor to elevated inflammation levels. The next chapter, "The Body Composition Challenge," will introduce you to the concept of body composition and losing the right kind of weight, or losing fat without losing any muscle. Throughout the rest of this book, we will teach you the most scientific, accurate, and effective methods to lose the most body fat and optimize your lean body mass. Your subsequent blood tests will confirm that the leaner you get, the better your blood results will be.

Chapter 6

The Body Composition Challenge

Obesity is not about excess weight; obesity is about excess fat.
—Michael L. Power, PhD, and Jay Schulkin, PhD,
The Evolution of Obesity, 2009

The Body Composition Challenge is *the* central challenge and *the* core issue of this book. All of the previous challenges we discussed boil down to this: How do we overcome all of the challenges we face and live in such a way that we lose fat while preserving and/or enhancing our lean body mass—so we actually become leaner, not just "thinner"?

When I first started my company in 1979, I did hydrostatic weighing, better known as the "dunk" test. I initially worked with a PhD in exercise physiology to learn exactly what body composition testing entailed and why it was so important. I then created a mobile testing unit that could test at every imaginable venue, including over 400 gyms and health clubs, 250 corporations, and 100 fire, police, and sheriff's departments. I tested hundreds of national and world-class athletes, plus dozens of sports teams.

We tested anywhere from twenty to one hundred clients a day. The client had to get into a tank of warm water in a swimsuit or two-piece. After months of testing and thousands of clients, we got so good we could estimate the person's body fat percentage within 1 percent. For a number of years, we tested all the senior swimmers and divers in a club called the Mission Viejo Nadadores every single month. I also did lectures on body composition and nutrition to the swimmers and divers, their parents, and their coaches. As a result of this association with the Nadadores, we tested most of the 1984 United States men's and women's Olympic swimming and diving team. I have also done a lot of work with Stanford University's men's swimming team. We learned that the leaner these athletes became, the better they performed and the healthier they got. This led to our current research and program, which focuses on teaching everyday people how they too, can optimize their body composition in an effort to become optimally healthy.

So what does body composition mean? Body composition means what percent of your total body weight is fat and what percent of your total body weight is lean body mass. Your fat weight is the total amount of fat in your body. Your lean body mass is your fat-free weight. Lean body mass includes your muscles, bones, organs, and fluids. Excess body fat for men is any body fat over 15 percent. Excess body fat for women is any body fat over 22 percent. Just as it's not healthy to have too much fat, it is not healthy to have too little muscle. Many women are under-muscled, even if they're thin. A thin, under-muscled woman is sometimes referred to as "skinny fat."

Why is body composition testing such a valuable tool? The challenge of losing weight is not as simple as "losing weight." The real challenge, the biological challenge, is losing the right *kind* of weight. The goal of losing weight is to optimize your body composition. Optimizing your body composition means enhancing your lean body mass (muscle) and only losing body fat. Ironically, your weight may or may not change. It is possible to get significantly leaner and not lose any weight at all, though most people will, in fact, lose weight (on the scale) too.

However, the reality is, your bathroom scale is just a small piece of the puzzle when it comes to getting lean. What you weigh on a scale does not really tell you much about the biological reality of your body or what kind of shape you are in. Just knowing someone's weight tells you nothing about their body, health, or fitness level. Why? Two people can weigh exactly the same, but be in very different levels of conditioning and fitness. One of these people can be in excellent shape; the other can be in awful shape.

I have worked with and personally tested the body fat of literally tens of thousands of people, including hundreds of world-class athletes. As an illustration of the fact that scale weight tells us virtually nothing about the health and fitness of a person, picture two women. Both of these women are exactly the same height: five feet, five inches tall. Both of these women weigh exactly the same: 138 pounds. Both women are exactly the same age: twenty-two. The first woman has the average body fat for an American woman: 36 percent. At 36 percent body fat and 138 pounds, this woman has 49.56 pounds of fat on her body and 88.44 pounds of lean body mass (muscle). The second woman is a world-class athlete (literally a world record holder). This world-class female athlete has 6.69 percent body fat. At 6.69 percent body fat and 138 pounds, this female athlete has only 9.13 pounds of fat on her body and she has 128.87 pounds of lean body mass (muscle). This world-class female athlete has literally forty pounds less fat in her body and forty pounds more muscle.

If you could see these two women in person, in two-piece swimsuits, side by side, the contrast would be striking. The first woman (36 percent fat) would look clearly (but not grossly) overweight. Her body is smooth and without tone or definition. She carries a lot of fat on the back of her arms, on her hips, and on her thighs. She has visible cellulite. The second woman (6.69 percent) is clearly a world-class athlete: lean, extremely fit-looking, and toned. She radiates health. She does *not* look skinny. She looks robustly and vigorously healthy. Yet, according to the scale, they appear the same.

The only strategy that has been proven to slow the aging process and prevent the physiological degradations associated with getting older is calorie restriction, or CR. Calorie restriction (CR) involves under-feeding your body without under-nourishing your body. The way we approach CR, however, takes this process one step further. We do not want you to restrict your calories indiscriminately, as most CR programs teach. The Joe Dillon Difference is not about getting thin, skinny, frail, or "dieting." The Joe Dillon Difference method of calorie restriction is about getting lean and eating in such a way that, although you are restricting your calories, you are still receiving all of your macronutrients, and each calorie you ingest contains the highest level of nutrition available. In other words, you want to get "the most bang for your buck" when it comes to nutrition. This distinction of determining what optimal nutrition truly looks like is crucial, and it is what sets us apart from those who talk about "dieting" or just restricting your calories indiscriminately.

The Challenge Ahead

Optimizing your body composition is a multi-factorial challenge. It involves confronting all of the factors that affect your body composition, including the mismatch between our evolutionary ideal and our modern environment. We live in an environment awash with easy calories and excess carbohydrates. Eating carbohydrates causes a spike in insulin (a hormone secreted by your pancreas) that in turn triggers your body's fat-storing mechanisms. As fat accumulates, especially in the abdominal region, it begins to emit dangerous inflammatory chemicals that contribute to disease development. Over time, after being constantly bombarded by insulin and high levels of blood sugar, your cells begin to resist insulin (they become insulin resistant), so your body works harder to produce more insulin while your blood sugar levels climb ever higher. This is the beginning stage of the metabolic disorder, which is closely linked to the development of diabetes and heart disease. The goal is to keep your levels of insulin and blood sugar constant.

Insulin resistance usually goes hand in hand with a sedentary lifestyle (lack of exercise). If you are not exercising at all, you cannot burn the optimal amount of fat—but if you are not exercising correctly, you will also not burn the optimal amount of fat, and you will not get lean. So learning how to exercise properly is the second challenge in obtaining ideal body composition.

Fat turns out to be hard to burn. Fat is also systemic, which means you cannot selectively reduce fat deposits (that means ab crunches burn zero fat). The technical term for fat burning is beta-oxidation. As the name implies, fat burning requires oxygen. It takes four to five times more oxygen to burn fat than it does to burn either sugar (carbohydrates) or muscle (protein). If you are puffing or panting when you exercise, you are not burning any fat, so high intensity exercise is not necessarily better. In fact, overtraining will actually waste away your lean body mass and make you fatter. If you want to reap the full reward of your workout, exercising in the optimal training heart rate range is crucial. We will teach you an ideal exercise to burn the optimal amount of body fat while building a significant amount of muscle. The more lean body mass you include in your aerobic exercise, the more calories and the more body fat you will burn.

Additionally, eating before and also immediately after your workout (a whey protein shake before and after your workout is the perfect meal) to preserve your lean mass (your muscles and bones) and to kick-start your recovery process, is crucial. Eating one more meal during your three-hour anabolic window is another factor in overcoming the body composition challenge. In fact, high levels of protein are essential to maintaining high levels of metabolically active lean muscle.

Lack of sleep, another challenge to becoming lean, will also make you fat, because your body will not be able to rebuild your muscle and because your body will release both insulin and cortisol. Insulin, remember, is the *most* powerful fat storing hormone in your body. Anything that raises insulin will make you fat (like lack sleep and chronic exhaustion). And excess cortisol will waste away your lean body mass *and* facilitate the storage of body fat (make you fatter). And last, but not least, it is crucial to stay well hydrated (drink enough water). Your muscles are 70 percent water.

What are the benefits of optimizing your body composition? Short term? Long term? We are assuming that one of the reasons you want to lose weight is that you would like to look better. More attractive. The most effective way to look better is to lower your body fat. Just losing weight indiscriminately (dieting) might make you look a little better in clothes. But optimizing your body composition (lowering your body fat while enhancing your lean body mass) will make you look good where and when you really want to look good: on the beach, at the pool, in bed. If you look good with little or no clothes on, you will look *great* with your clothes on. It is a win/win. By doing what you need to do to optimize your body composition, you will automatically become more fit, more toned, and radiantly healthy. By optimizing your body composition, in the short term, you will look great and feel great.

In the long term, optimizing your body composition will significantly improve your health and slow the aging process. Excess body fat is a high-risk physiological marker for chronic inflammation, which has been linked with everything from diabetes to heart disease to Alzheimer's. Getting your body fat as low as you can while staying within the healthy ranges set by exercise physiological research for most athletes (world-class athletes are genetic exceptions) of any age (6–12 percent for men and 12–18 percent for women) will make you exceptionally healthy and help you age the most successfully. By getting and staying lean, you will look and feel more youthful right through middle-age and well into your golden years.

For all practical purposes, you can't get too lean. Reducing your body fat is a self-limiting process. The leaner you get, the harder it gets to get any leaner. The leaner you get, the healthier you are. All the things you need to do in order to get lean will only make you robustly healthy. For in order to get lean, you have to enhance your lean body mass and you have to burn fat. So you will end up strong and functional, and in great shape. You *cannot* diet yourself lean. Getting leaner is a dynamic process that involves the interaction of eating a highly nutritious, well-balanced diet; getting an optimal amount of full-body aerobic exercise; drinking a generous amount of water; taking pharmaceutical-grade supplements; and getting optimal amounts of sleep.

In the next section, we will address the Biological Essentials necessary to most effectively optimize your body composition to give you a body you are proud of, even with the lights on and even with your clothes off. And to sweeten the bargain, remember: You will have the best blood panel you have ever had in your life, and you will get into your best aerobic shape ever (giving you tremendous energy and confidence). So now that you are aware of the challenges you face, it's time to find the solutions.

Section Two

Biological Essentials

Chapter 7

Biological Essential: Oxygen

How long can you hold your breath?
                                                    —Joe Dillon

From this point forward, we will progress from challenges to the resolution of our challenges. There are six major challenges you will confront every day for the rest of your life: evolution, development, environment, aging, inflammation, and body composition. These six challenges are your biological reality. Now, let's look at the biological essentials that each of us *must* have and begin to discuss how we can best resolve our challenges in such a way as to lose weight most effectively.

Health is molecular and genetic. This means that our bodies require specific biologic molecules or processes in order to promote optimal gene expression. In order of importance, the eight Biological Essentials are: oxygen, water, the eight essential amino acids, the two essential fats, low glycemic load carbohydrates, full-body aerobic exercise, optimal sleep, and optimal amounts of micronutrients, such as vitamin C. Everything we do up-regulates or down-regulates the expression of particular genes or sets of genes. For optimal gene expression, and therefore optimal health, we need to do eight fundamental and essential things.

The first Biological Essential we are going to discuss is oxygen. In this chapter, we will start with deep evolutionary time and discuss how our oxygen-rich atmosphere came about; how living organisms made radical changes to cope with and exploit the addition of oxygen to our world; how and why oxygen respiration is an evolutionary advantage; and why oxygen respiration is conserved to this day.

Beginning in deep evolutionary time, for over one billion years after the earth was formed more than 4.6 billion years ago, the atmosphere of our earth had virtually no oxygen. Approximately 3.5 billion years ago, when the very earliest single-cell organisms appeared, they were all anaerobic, meaning their metabolisms did not need oxygen. Some of these simple cells were photosynthesizing cyanobacteria. Photosynthesis is the process by which these bacteria captured energy from the sun in the form of photons and converted it into chemical energy. All plants use photosynthesis to this day. In fact, life on our planet could not exist without photosynthesis. These cyanobacteria used water as a reducing agent and produced oxygen as a waste product. As a result, the oxygen concentration in our earth's atmosphere slowly began to rise.

If we had cyanobacteria producing free oxygen as a waste product, why didn't we quickly have an oxygen-rich atmosphere? Because oxygen is an electron hog. There are only four electrons in its outer electron shell, which can hold up to eight electrons. As a result, oxygen has a ravenous hunger to bind with, or oxidize, nearly anything it comes in contact with. As a result of this powerful and fundamental property of oxygen, all the free oxygen the cyanobacteria produced instantly combined with iron to form iron oxide. Accordingly, it took over a billion years, from approximately 3.5 billion years ago to 2.41 billion years ago, for all the available iron to become oxygen saturated. Finally, from 2.41 billion years ago to 2.32 billion years ago, free oxygen began to accumulate fast enough to trigger what is known as the Great Oxygen Event.

The Great Oxygen Event triggered profound changes in our earth's atmosphere and in living organisms. First, the rise in free oxygen was toxic to many of the existing anaerobic organisms. As a result, about 99 percent of all anaerobic organisms went extinct. Photosynthesizing cyanobacteria, however, were able to adapt. In fact, the chloroplasts (the organelles where photosynthesis takes place) in every plant are actually cyanobacteria that were incorporated into plant cells hundreds of millions of years ago.

As part of the evolutionary process, those organisms, which were better suited for the new oxygen atmosphere, thrived and new organisms appeared.

These new organisms were aerobic, which meant they required oxygen to perform life processes. To this day, virtually all living animals, including human beings, use aerobic metabolism. As part of the evolutionary adaptation to the Great Oxygen Event, the eukaryotic cell appeared. A eukaryotic cell is a complex cell with a nucleus and other organelles. And along with the eukaryotic cell came the appearance of mitochondria. Mitochondria are the organelles in every single one of the cells in your body where aerobic metabolism takes place (Alberts et al 2008).

The Great Oxygen Event led to an increase in free oxygen, which also caused an increase of ozone (O_3) and the formation of the ozone layer. The ozone layer was crucially important to protect land organisms from the damaging effect of the sun's powerful radiation.

Between 700 million years ago and 540 million years ago, the amount of free oxygen in our earth's atmosphere surged again. This surge led to what is known as the Cambrian Explosion. At this point, the amount of free oxygen in the earth's atmosphere had climbed significantly. The Cambrian Explosion is the greatest explosion of biological diversity in history. The precursors for virtually all of the plants and animals we see today evolved during the Cambrian Explosion, including the very earliest mammals. The oxygen content of our earth's atmosphere continued to rise, until it peaked at about 35 percent about 300 million years ago. There was so much oxygen and the atmosphere of our earth was so dense that it enabled the growth of huge insects. For example, dragonflies had wing spans of 2.5 feet. Eventually, the atmosphere settled back down to approximately 21 percent, as it is today.

Now that we know this change took place, why did aerobic organisms continue to thrive and multiply, while anaerobic organisms became extinct? What is the evolutionary advantage of aerobic metabolism versus anaerobic metabolism? And why was aerobic metabolism evolutionarily conserved? It all comes down to energy. Cellular metabolism, whether aerobic or anaerobic, is the process of converting food molecules, like glucose, to carbon dioxide and water. The unit of energy currency in all living things is a molecule called ATP (adenosine triphosphate). With anaerobic metabolism, each molecule of glucose only yields two molecules of ATP, whereas with aerobic metabolism, every molecule of glucose yields thirty-six molecules of ATP. Therefore, aerobic metabolism is eighteen times more energy efficient than anaerobic metabolism. When evolution finds something that works, it keeps or conserves it. The fundamental processes of our metabolism are hundreds of millions of years old.

Oxygen was first independently discovered by a Swedish chemist, Carl Wilhelm Scheele, in 1772, and by an English chemist Joseph Priestly in 1774. Priestly published first in 1774 and is often given credit for the initial discovery of oxygen. Antoine Lavoisier, a French scientist, was the first to recognize oxygen as a pure element between 1775 and 1780. Lavoisier also invented the name oxygen and explained combustion as a chemical reaction between oxygen and the material being burned. Today, our atmosphere is composed of approximately 21 percent (20.8 percent) oxygen. Oxygen comes in a package of two oxygen atoms bonded together. This common form of free oxygen is called dioxygen or O_2.

Turning to the present, what is the structure and function of oxygen in our body right now? Just as water moves from the sky to earth and back, oxygen is also cycled through our environment. Plants, including algae, and many bacteria represent the beginning of the oxygen cycle. As we learned, plants use the energy of the sun (photons) to convert carbon dioxide and water into carbohydrates and oxygen in a process called photosynthesis. Think of plants as breathing in carbon dioxide and breathing out oxygen. Animals are the other half of the oxygen cycle. We breathe in oxygen that we use to break down carbohydrates into energy (ATP) in a metabolic process called cellular respiration. Cellular metabolism or respiration takes place in the mitochondria of our cells. Carbon dioxide produced during respiration is breathed out.

Moving from a cellular perspective to the perspective of our entire body, we have a system designed to transport oxygen from the point where we breathe it into our lungs which circulates it out to every single cell in our body. This system is called our cardiovascular system. Our cardiovascular system is composed of our heart, our lungs, and our entire circulatory system. We breathe oxygen into our lungs. This oxygen is picked up by red blood cells. Red blood cells contain an iron-rich compound called hemoglobin. Our heart pumps our blood from our lungs through our arteries out to our body. Our trillions of red blood cells (approximately twenty to thirty trillion) carry oxygen to every single one of our cells. The oxygen is dropped off and carbon dioxide (the waste product of cellular respiration) is picked up and pumped back through our veins to our heart and lungs, where we exhale the carbon dioxide out into the atmosphere.

The key to energy is having a strong, efficient cardiovascular system. If you want to have more energy, you have to have a stronger heart. If you want more energy, you want to do everything you can to enhance your cardiovascular system. Energy is a simple equation: More oxygen equals more energy. Which human beings have the greatest amount of energy? World- class aerobic athletes like cross-country skiers, rowers, or marathon runners. What is one thing all these athletes have in common? A very low resting heart rate, which means they have very strong hearts. Your body does not lie.

Lack of oxygen is called hypoxia. You experience hypoxia when you try to swim under water. After a fairly short time, you get this very insistent urge to come up and take a breath. Why? Partly because the oxygen content in your blood is dropping, but primarily because the level of carbon dioxide is rapidly rising. Homeostasis is your body's effort to keep your biological parameters within optimal ranges. You have genetically built into your body these optimal ranges and ratios for all kinds of things. The optimal oxygen/carbon dioxide ratio of your blood is crucial to your brain and to staying alive. The oxygen/carbon dioxide ratio of your blood is a critical biomarker. When the carbon dioxide content of your blood gets too high relative to the oxygen content of your blood, you begin to get intense messages to breathe.

Hypoxia is also why most people cannot live on the top of Mount Everest. At twenty-nine thousand feet, at an altitude called the death zone, we cannot breathe in enough oxygen to support human life (Beall 2006). It is not that there is not enough oxygen. The percent of the atmosphere that is oxygen is the same as at sea level. What is different is the air pressure. The air pressure on top of Mount Everest is only 33 percent of the air pressure at sea level. As a result, there is not enough air pressure to "push" the oxygen into our cells, so we can't breathe in enough oxygen to stay alive.

We don't have to climb to the top of Mount Everest to feel a change in air pressure and therefore feel difficulty getting enough oxygen. Ascending to even seventy-three hundred feet altitude can make a big difference. Common symptoms of sudden ascent can include headache, nausea, weakness or fatigue, dizziness or lightheadedness, and difficulty sleeping. And altitude can affect performance. The impact of high altitude on athletic performance was clearly demonstrated at the 1968 Summer Olympic Games held at Mexico City. Athletes who lived and trained at sea level turned out to be at a major disadvantage, especially in events that involved endurance or stamina.

The contrast between athletes who lived and trained at sea levels and athletes who lived and trained at altitude was graphically clear in distance running events. The Mexico City Olympic Games in 1968 marked the emergence of the Kenyans as distance runners. Kenyan runners live and train at between eight thousand and eleven thousand feet altitude. When they ran at the seventy-three-hundred-foot altitude of Mexico City, the Kenyans were already fully acclimated. Runners who lived and trained at sea level were gasping for air and could not compete with the Kenyans. This was the beginning of distance runners worldwide doing at least some of their training at high altitude. Marathon runners like Frank Shorter moved to places like Boulder, Colorado, at fifty-four hundred feet altitude and other locations where they could run at altitudes as high as ten thousand or twelve thousand feet. Four years later, Frank Shorter won the gold medal in the marathon at the 1972 Olympics held at sea level in Munich, Germany.

When the Kenyans dominated all the distance events at the Mexico City Olympics, exercise physiology researchers wanted to understand exactly why. It turns out that the human body can make a number of adjustments, if given enough time to acclimate, so we can function at nearly the same level of performance as we did at sea level. Some of the keys are to give our body enough time to adjust and not try to do too much, too soon. As part of this physiological adjustment or acclimatization, our body increases the number of red blood cells and our hemoglobin becomes richer. All of these adjustments allow our body to get more oxygen, despite the lower air pressure of higher altitudes. But it takes time. Weeks and months. And we will never be 100 percent acclimated. Plus we lose it very quickly once we descend back to sea level.

Now that we understand the importance of maximizing oxygen availability, how can we manage our environments to ensure this? The first thing to avoid is smoking. Nothing interferes with your body's ability to carry oxygen more than smoking of any kind. Smoking is devastating to your body. If a pregnant woman smokes, she is depriving her fetus of precious oxygen. Under low oxygen conditions, as you learned, the fetus must conserve oxygen, creating all sorts of problems for the fetus later in life. Smoking may even cause mental retardation or some level of decreased brain functionality, for as the fetus makes "difficult" decisions as to where to distribute this limited supply of oxygen, its brain may not get enough precious oxygen for full development. Other organs will also pay a price for this oxygen deprivation.

Secondhand smoke is also damaging to both children and adults. Smoking in a house or a car with children compromises the development of those children for life. Never have children in any kind of closed environment with smoke of any kind (cigarette, cigar, or pipe).

When it comes to the Aging Challenge, oxygen is a two-edged sword. On the one hand, we should strive to stay in the best aerobic shape we can as this is paramount to minimizing the effects of aging. Aerobic conditioning is *the key* to energy and functionality, and aerobic fitness is the one thing that has been proven to create neurogenesis (the creation of new brain cells).

On the other hand, oxygen is a very "high maintenance" molecule and if not treated properly, can also be very harmful. When the Great Oxygen Event took place, it meant mass extinction for anaerobic organisms. One of the reasons for this is that oxygen, particularly in a form called reactive oxygen species or ROS—also known as free radicals or singlet oxygen—is dangerous and toxic. To protect against ROS, aerobic organisms quickly developed molecules to neutralize this toxic form of oxygen. These molecules are called antioxidants. However, as you age, and even more so if you are overweight, your endogenous (internal) antioxidants become diminished and/or they become less effective.

At the same time, as you age, and again, especially if you are overweight, you actually produce *more* free radicals. Also, because our current low quality food supply has severely compromised levels of antioxidants in our diets, we are not ingesting nearly the level of high quality antioxidants we ingested in hunter-gatherer times. These factors—increased free radicals and reduced antioxidants—hinder our ability to neutralize these toxic molecules. And as we mentioned, oxygen is an electron hog. So when an oxygen molecule is missing even one electron, it has a voracious appetite to bind with anything it can to pick up that missing electron. One of the most common examples of this is rust. If the free radical oxygen binds with iron, it is called iron oxide, or rust. Rust destroys iron.

This happens within the human body as well. One prominent theory of aging is called the free radical theory of aging, or the "rusting" of the body by free radical oxygen. Free radical oxygen also contributes to chronic inflammation. This is why one of the healthiest things we can do is to take antioxidants such as vitamin C and vitamin E. Antioxidants are known as free-radical scavengers because they neutralize electron-hungry oxygen molecules by donating an electron. We will talk more about antioxidants and other beneficial supplements in our chapter on Supplementation.

And now for the most important question in this chapter: Why is oxygen such an important factor in the resolution of the Body Composition Challenge and losing weight? As we mentioned, the technical name for fat burning is beta-oxidation. Beta-oxidation, or fat burning, requires oxygen. In fact, body fat is hard to burn. Body fat requires four to five times more oxygen to be burned or oxidized than either carbohydrates or proteins. So the more oxygen you can supply to your body, the more efficiently and effectively you can burn fat. *The* key to getting more oxygen to your cells and the hundreds of fat-burning mitochondria in each of your cells is a strong, efficient cardiovascular system: your heart, your lungs, and your circulatory system.

But just like getting lean, fat burning is self-limiting. There is a threshold, called your anaerobic threshold, above which the amount of fat your body burns during exercise decreases drastically. If you want to burn the most fat when you exercise, you must involve the greatest amount of lean body mass in your aerobic exercise and work at a pace where you can breathe comfortably. And you want the greatest number of mitochondria in each of your muscle cells because this is where beta-oxidation takes place. We will teach you just such an exercise.

You also want to avoid anything that might interfere with your body's ability to burn fat. This includes fat in your bloodstream. This fat may come directly from a high-fat diet. Or, it may come from eating too many carbohydrates, which the hormone insulin converts to triglycerides (blood fat).

Excess blood fat makes the outside of your red blood cells sticky. When these sticky red blood cells bump into each other (which they are doing all the time), they stick together and form clumps. A capillary (a microscopic blood vessel) is only large enough for *one* red blood cell to pass through at a time. This tight fit between the red blood cell and the walls of the capillaries allows the oxygen/carbon dioxide exchange to take place (the oxygen is dropped off at the cell and the waste product of cellular respiration, carbon dioxide, is picked up and carried back to the lungs to be exhaled out). Clumps of red blood cells stuck together cannot fit through a capillary. Instead, they get stuck, like in a traffic jam, at the forks where the capillary is only one red blood cell wide. The end result? Your ability to carry oxygen is reduced by as much as 30 to 40 percent after a high-fat and/or high-carbohydrate meal. This is one reason you feel sleepy or tired after a heavy meal. Your brain is not getting enough oxygen. Sleepiness after any meal is an indicator you have eaten too many carbs and/or too much food in that meal. Your body does not lie.

But don't worry—we have developed a scientifically based method to maximize the level of oxygen in your blood so you have the most energy, the greatest mental clarity, and burn the most fat.

Chapter 8

Biological Essential: Water

Just because it's wet, doesn't mean it will hydrate you.
—Joe Dillon

When our earth first came into being 4.6 billion years ago, it was a fiery, molten ball. There was water vapor in the atmosphere, but the surface of our earth was too hot for the water vapor to become liquid. It took about 500–600 million years for the surface of our earth to cool enough for the water vapor in the atmosphere to condense into liquid water. When our earth was about four billion years old, the true hydrosphere developed, and with it came the water cycle and the beginning of life.

The hydrosphere is often called the water sphere because it contains all of the earth's water found in the oceans, glaciers, streams, lakes, the soil, groundwater, and in the air. The hydrosphere interacts with, and is influenced by, all the other earth's spheres. The water in the hydrosphere is distributed among the other spheres, meaning that water is held in oceans, lakes and streams at the surface of the earth. Water is also found in vapor, liquid, and solid states in the earth's atmosphere. The biosphere (all living organisms) serves as an interface between the hydrosphere, the lithosphere (the solid, rocky crust covering the surface of the planet), and the atmosphere, which is accomplished by plant transpiration (the release of water into the atmosphere by plants).

Water is a limited and recycled resource. Water is used over and over again and has been for billions of years. The water cycle describes the continuous movement of water from the ocean to the air and land, and then back to the ocean. The sun, which drives the water cycle, heats water in the oceans and seas. Water evaporates from the oceans as vapor and, once in the air, changes from a liquid to a gas. Water also evaporates from plants and the soil. In the process of evaporation, water is purified. Also in the process of evaporation, water takes up energy from the surroundings and cools the environment. As the water vapor in the atmosphere cools, it condenses into liquid droplets. These droplets grow and combine until they are too heavy and fall back to the earth as liquid rain, solid ice (hail), or snow. Water is temporarily stored in lakes, glaciers, underground, or in living organisms, which use it for innumerable life processes. Over time, the water moves from these places through streams and rivers and is returned to the ocean.

Water can exist in three states: liquid (water is liquid under usual conditions); solid (ice); and gas (water vapor in the atmosphere). Liquid water covers about 70 percent of our earth's surface and is vital to all forms of life. Clean, fresh drinking water is essential to human beings and all other life forms.

What is water exactly? Water is a chemical substance with the chemical formula H_2O, meaning that a molecule of water contains one atom of oxygen and two atoms of hydrogen. All the atoms in a water molecule are connected by covalent bonds. A water molecule is not a linear molecule, however. Electrically, water is a polar molecule, meaning that water is slightly negative on the oxygen end and slightly positive on the hydrogen end. Because of this polarity, water can form an unusually large number of intermolecular hydrogen bonds for a molecule its size. Water is also a good solvent. In fact, water is often referred to as the universal solvent. Examples of substances that dissolve in water include salts, sugars, acids, alkalis, and some gases, especially oxygen and carbon dioxide (carbonated water). All the major components of our body's cells are dissolved in water, including proteins, DNA, and polysaccharides (simple and complex sugars).

From a biological standpoint, water has many properties that are critical for the proliferation of life. Water allows organic compounds to react in ways that ultimately allow replication. Water is vital both as a solvent, in which many of the body's solutes are dissolved, and as an essential part of many of the metabolic processes within our body. Metabolism is the sum total of anabolism and catabolism. In anabolism, water is removed from molecules (through energy that requires enzymatic chemical reactions) in order to grow larger molecules (for example: starches, triglycerides, and proteins for storage of fuels and information). In catabolism, water is used to break bonds in order to generate smaller molecules (for example, glucose, fatty acids and amino acids to be used for fuels for energy use or other purposes). These particular metabolic processes could not exist without water.

Water makes up 70 percent of your body and is essential. To show how connected our bodies are to the earth, it is no coincidence that the earth is 70 percent water and our bodies are also 70 percent water. Water is involved in every function of your body. Water helps transport nutrients and waste products in and out of cells. Water is necessary for all digestive, absorption, circulatory, and excretory functions. Water is essential for the utilization of water-soluble vitamins. Water is also essential for the maintenance of proper body temperature (sweating, for example). Water is crucial for muscle tone as 70 percent of your muscles are water. Water is your body's number one detoxifier.

To further underscore how essential water is to life and to the health of your body, let's see what happens when your body is deprived of water. As you may know, we humans can go for many weeks without any food. But in less than one week without water, we will die, even in a temperate climate. The condition we are describing is dehydration. What are some of the symptoms of dehydration?

Like many things in your body, our fluid levels are dynamic. When your fluid intake does not replenish your fluid loss, dehydration results. Research has found that 75 percent of all Americans are chronically dehydrated. Unfortunately, because many people's thirst mechanism is so weak, it is often mistaken for hunger. Eating when you are actually thirsty increases dehydration.

There are degrees of dehydration. Symptoms of mild dehydration (1 percent to 2 percent water loss) include restlessness or irritability, sunken eyes, dry mouth and tongue, thirsty, abnormally dark urine, headache, nausea, and dizziness upon standing up.

As a person becomes more dehydrated, their blood plasma volume decreases and their blood pressure drops. To compensate for these physiological changes, the person's heart rate speeds up and they breathe at a faster rate. With decreased sweating, their body temperature rises. They may become groggy, have severe cramps, and become delirious. All these consequences are the direct result of the person not drinking enough water.

Of course, many factors contribute to the onset of dehydration. Exercise, particularly in the heat, can be dehydrating. Alcohol is dehydrating. In fact, the number one cause of hangovers is dehydration. Caffeine and prescription drugs are also dehydrating. Sugar and refined carbohydrates are dehydrating. Salt is dehydrating, but salt is a two-edged sword. All human beings need some salt (sodium chloride), but most people consume excessive amounts of salt. Processed foods tend to be extremely salty. Eating salty foods and then washing them down with sugary soda only compounds the problem of dehydration. Many people do not drink anything that is truly hydrating, which is why most people are chronically dehydrated their entire lives. Remember my quote, "Just because it's wet, doesn't mean it will hydrate you."

One of the most informative biomarkers to observe is the color of your urine. Your urine should be clear to a light yellow color. It is very simple. When your urine gets darker than this, you are falling behind the fluid dynamic curve, and it is time to drink some pure water (American College of Sports Medicine 2011).

When it comes to energy and performance, even mild dehydration can be devastating. As little as 1–2 percent dehydration can reduce your endurance by 20–30 percent. Your core temperature will climb. Your perceived exertion (how hard the exercise feels to you) will get harder and harder (McArdle et al 2009).

As we get older, our sensation of thirst diminishes even more. Chronic dehydration becomes an even bigger issue. Optimal hydration is kind of like optimal sleep as we get older. We still need just as much. It just becomes more of a challenge to get it. In fact, dehydration as we age is such a problem that the number one cause of memory loss in older people is dehydration.

And now for the key question: What does drinking water and staying well hydrated have to do with losing weight? It turns out that drinking pure water, and lots of it, is the single most important catalyst in losing weight and keeping it off. Water suppresses your appetite naturally and helps your body metabolize stored fat. Your kidneys cannot function without an abundant supply of pure water. If you don't drink enough water, your kidneys cannot work to capacity. If your kidneys cannot work to capacity, some of your kidney's load is dumped on your liver. One of your liver's primary functions is to metabolize stored fat into usable energy. But if your liver has to do some of your kidney's work, your liver is compromised. As a result, your liver metabolizes less fat and weight loss stops. To keep your kidneys working at an optimal level, drink at least 8–12, eight-ounce glasses of pure water every day, spread throughout your day. Sixteen eight-ounce glasses of pure water per day is even better.

Drinking an optimal amount of water every day is also the most effective way to eliminate fluid retention. Your body can be contrary. If you deprive your body of something it needs, your body perceives that deprivation as a threat to its survival. If you don't drink enough water, your body will hang on to every drop. This is why diuretics for weight loss are a quick fix that ultimately makes the problem worse. It may seem counterintuitive, but if you want your body to let go of retained fluid, drink a lot of pure water. The same concept holds true for food.

Skipping meals will make you fat, as your body perceives lack of food as a potential famine and hangs on to every pound (Davy 2010).

If water is so essential, what counts toward your water intake and what does not count? The following is a list of excellent sources of water (prioritized in descending order from the most pure down, according to the National Science Foundation 2011):

- **Distilled water**.

- **Filtered water**. Reverse osmosis is the best of the filtered but any filter will do, even a filter on the tap in your kitchen.

- **Bottled water**.

- **Carbonated water**.

- **Herbal tea, decaf coffee, and decaf tea** if unsweetened and made with pure water.

- **Tap water**. Tap water contains chlorine so it is best to fill a pitcher of tap water and put it in your refrigerator. All the chlorine will gas off with a few hours.

What does *not* count toward your water intake?

- **Alcohol** (of any kind). Alcohol is a major dehydrator.

- **Juice** (of any kind). All juice is pure sugar and therefore a major dehydrator.

- **Sodas** (of any kind). Sodas are all major dehydrators.

- **Many sports drinks**. Many sports drinks have the same sugar content as sodas and are therefore dehydrators.

- **Coffee** (caffeinated). Caffeine is a major dehydrator.

To calculate the optimal amount of water for your body, take your total body weight and divide it in half. That is the optimal number of ounces of pure water your body needs every day. For example, a two hundred–pound person needs approximately one hundred ounces of pure water every day. One hundred ounces is 12.5 eight-ounce glasses of pure water. This is a general guideline. Pregnant and lactating women need 50 percent more water. Exercising athletes, particularly if the weather is hot, will need significantly more water. Listen to *your* body.

Getting and staying well hydrated is a habit. Stock your house up with cases of water. Have water in plain sight in your kitchen. Have water in your car. Have water in sight and within arm's reach wherever you work. Get in the habit of drinking a glass of water *before* every meal. Drink lots of water *with* every meal. You will get full sooner. You will feel more satisfied. And lots of water actually helps your body digest your food.

As with our first Biological Essential, oxygen, we want to do everything we can to get and stay well hydrated, and we want to avoid things that dehydrate our body. The choice is yours. You can make a difference. Why not start now?

Chapter 9

Biological Essential: Lean Protein

Meat makes us human.
—Henry T. Bunn, PhD,
Evolution of the Human Diet, 2006

Like oxygen and water, the third Biological Essential, lean protein, is deeply ingrained in our DNA.

Proteins were the very first organic molecules, and some of the earliest organic molecules were informational proteins, namely RNA (ribonucleic acid). Over time, an even more effective organic molecule for transmitting genetic information called DNA (deoxyribonucleic acid) replaced RNA as the primary informational molecule.

As of today, DNA is present in every cell in your body and responds to your lifestyle. Your genes are constantly being turned on and off depending upon what you eat, how much sleep you get, whether you exercise or not, and your stress levels, just to name a few behaviors. Genes in turn dictate the synthesis of proteins from amino acids. There are eight *essential* amino acids, which your genes use to synthesize twenty principle proteins. From these twenty proteins, your body synthesizes literally thousands of different kinds of proteins. Proteins are the workhorses of the human body. Nothing biological happens in your body without protein being involved in some fundamental way.

In human health, we are primarily concerned with the eight *essential* amino acids. The concept of *essential* means that our bodies must have these eight amino acids, yet we cannot synthesize them. Therefore, we must ingest (eat) these eight essential amino acids. We cannot store protein, so we have to eat the eight essential amino acids every three to five hours. The single best source of these eight crucial amino acids is lean, complete protein.

Expanding upon our evolutionary story of protein, it turns out that protein had a huge impact on our development as modern *Homo sapiens*. The first fundamental separation of us from our common ancestor with apes was our ability to walk on two legs. That split from a common ancestor took place roughly six to eight million years ago. The next major step down the evolutionary road was the invention of tools, which occurred about 2.6 million years ago (Johanson 2009). Not only was this literally the birth of all human technology, but the invention of tools also had a profound impact on the development of our brain.

Our big, complex, highly intelligent brains are the single biggest difference between human beings and all other organisms on the earth. But our big brains are extremely high maintenance organs (Aiello and Wheeler 1995). Your brain requires—in fact, demands—an extremely high level of oxygen and nutritional support. And this is where tools become so important. Our very earliest bipedal ancestors were small (about three feet tall), had small brains (about the size of an orange), and were primarily vegetarian. This did not change for millions of years. Then there was a split in the family tree. One branch became more specialized vegetarians with huge back teeth for grinding coarse vegetable matter. That branch eventually became extinct. The other branch invented tools and later evolved into *Homo sapiens*.

The very first tools were crude, no more than broken rocks. But the archaeological evidence clearly shows that these rocks were broken in very specific ways to achieve a sharp cutting edge. The raw material to make these early tools had been carefully and deliberately chosen. The raw material had also been carried a long distance from its volcanic source to the place where the tools were made. The most effective tools were made from rocks such as chert or obsidian, which when struck in a certain way with a hammer-stone formed a particularly sharp and serrated edge.

What is the significance of sharp-edged stones to the evolutionary development of the human brain? With these newly invented sharp-edged stones, our early ancestors could, for the very first time, butcher carcasses that had been deserted by the larger predators of that prehistoric era (saber-toothed cats, leopards, and hyenas, for example). Prior to this, our ancestors could not get through the thick, tough hide of an antelope, for example, with just their fingers. Now they could cut through the hide, and shear off hunks of extremely nutrient-dense meat. They could also smash the bones and skull and extract the fatty, nutrient-rich marrow and brain. Both the meat and the bone marrow of these wild animals were not only rich in protein, but also in an essential fat called omega-3.

Lean, complete protein (that is, protein containing all eight essential amino acids) and essential omega-3 fat are the ultimate brain foods. As a result, over time, our ancestors' brains began to grow and evolve. This became a feed-forward loop. As our ancestors' diets improved, and their brains grew bigger and smarter, our ancestors evolved from opportunistic scavengers into skillful, effective hunters. As our ancestors' hunting skills increased, so did the proportion of meat in their diets. With more and more high quality protein and essential fat, our ancestors not only grew bigger, smarter brains, they grew in stature from around three feet tall to over six feet tall. This took hundreds of thousands of years.

Our hunter-gatherer ancestors were incredibly healthy, with none of the degenerative diseases that plague modern man today. The size and health of human beings peaked at about ten to twelve thousand years ago, with the advent of the agricultural revolution. The agricultural revolution was a negative watershed moment in human history from the perspective of health. With the agricultural revolution came a fundamental shift in the human diet from a meat-based, high-protein, moderate-healthy-fat, totally unprocessed low-carbohydrate diet to a sugar-based diet based on cereal grains (Lindeberg 2010). And with that fundamental dietary shift came the arrival of degenerative disease. The shift was slow at first, but in the last thirty years it has reached epidemic global proportions, with no let-up in sight.

From a developmental point of view, the nine months a fetus spends in its mother's womb and the six to twelve months a baby breastfeeds are crucial to the developing metabolism, future health, and risk of degenerative disease. Because the nine-month gestation and breastfeeding are so critical to the survival and long-term health of the child, pregnant and lactating mothers need 50 percent more protein and 50 percent more essential fat. These biological essentials are crucial to the restoration of the health of the mother and to the growth and the development of the child, especially its rapidly growing brain.

On the other hand, we live in an extremely unhealthy environment. In fact, our environment is so unhealthy it is literally obesogenic, meaning that our environment and culture encourages obesity and degenerative disease. As a result of America's obesogenic environment, the average American eats over 150 pounds of sugar a year. Over 90 percent of all Americans are woefully deficient in both protein and essential fat. Seventy-five percent of all Americans are chronically dehydrated. Those of us who actually care about our health have to work conscientiously if we want to get optimal amounts of the eight essential amino acids and essential omega-3 fat in our daily diets.

The Aging Challenge is characterized by loss: loss of strength, loss of energy, and loss of lean body mass (sarcopenia). Loss of control over our blood sugar levels, and therefore our insulin levels, is also characteristic of the Aging Challenge. As a result, eating an optimal amount of lean, complete protein becomes paramount as we age. As we age, however, most people have a much more difficult time assimilating the essential nutrients. Our losing battle with the Inflammation Challenge is an added insult. A high intake of lean, complete protein is essential to our ongoing efforts to control our inflammation markers, especially insulin.

The Inflammation Challenge is present at every age, even in the womb. Central to controlling inflammation is controlling blood sugar levels and insulin levels. Lean, complete protein is the cornerstone to the nutritional control of both blood sugar and insulin and therefore inflammation.

The most effective sources of the eight essential amino acids are lean, complete proteins. But what, exactly, are lean, complete proteins? The definition of a lean protein is a protein source that contains no more than 20 percent of its calories as fat. This is an important distinction, because conventional wisdom encourages us to think of foods like beef steak as a good protein source. In reality, a typical steak contains more than 75 percent of its calories as fat. Now, on the package label, you will probably see a very different number.

Whenever you see a fat percentage on a food label, it means what percent of the *weight* of that food is fat. Fat floats. Fat is not very dense weight-wise. So this is deliberately misleading. A much more accurate depiction of the fat content of a given food is what percent of the *calories* are fat. With a very simple formula you can easily calculate what percent of the calories of a given food, or, in this case, protein, is fat. Simply take the grams of fat per serving and multiply that by nine. Why nine? One gram of carbohydrate contains four calories. One gram of protein contains four calories. And one gram of fat contains nine calories. So by multiplying the grams of fat per serving times nine, we are converting the grams of fat to calories of fat. Then take the product of the multiplication of the grams of fat times nine and divide that by the total calories per serving. The result is the percent of total calories as fat.

Consider extra lean hamburger. The label says it contains no more than 15 percent fat. One hundred grams of extra lean hamburger contains fifteen grams of fat, or 15 percent. But that is not the true picture. One hundred grams (3.5 ounces) of extra lean hamburger contains 215 calories. So, if you take the fifteen grams of fat times nine calories per gram of fat, you will see that this equals 135 calories of fat. Now divide 135 calories of fat by 215 calories per serving, and we get 63 percent. This means that 63 percent of all the calories in the extra lean hamburger are pure fat, mostly saturated fat. This is empirical proof that extra lean hamburger is *not* a lean protein. Extra lean hamburger is a high-fat food and just another example of the Black Box of Conventional Wisdom (marketing) misleading us.

A short list of examples of truly lean proteins includes foods like white and dark turkey meat (no skin), wild game meat (tenderloins and medallions only), the white meat of chicken (no dark meat or skin), fish, egg whites (zero fat), and whey protein isolate (zero fat).

Now that you have a clearer understanding of what lean means, what does complete mean? As you've learned, there are eight essential amino acids. A complete protein is a protein that contains *all* eight essential amino acids. For the record, there are no truly complete proteins in the plant world. The only truly complete proteins are found in the animal world. This is one reason a strict vegetarian diet is not healthy. A lacto-ovo vegetarian can get by, but not a strict vegan.

What are the benefits of eating the eight essential amino acids and lean, complete protein? The biological reality of your body is that there is only one thing on the earth that can build muscles, bones, and heart muscle: lean, complete protein. You can't build muscles and bones with donuts. In fact, sugar blocks protein synthesis. Virtually every important biological component of your body is made out of amino acids (protein): muscles, bones, enzymes, hormones, ligaments, tendons, and even the hemoglobin in every one of the trillions of red blood cells that allows you to carry oxygen. Proteins are the workhorses of the human body. Proteins are actively involved in virtually every metabolic process.

And now for our central question: What does lean, complete protein have to do with losing weight? After staying well hydrated, keeping your blood sugar stable is the next most critical step to effectively losing weight (fat). The key to controlling your blood sugar levels is controlling the hormone insulin. The hormone insulin (which, by the way, is a protein) is the most powerful fat storing hormone in the human body. Lean, complete protein is crucial to managing insulin and keeping your blood sugar stable. That is why the cornerstone of every single meal is a fist-sized portion of lean, complete protein. Make a fist. The volume of your fist is approximately the amount of lean, complete protein you need to put into your body at the start of *every* single meal. We recommend that you eat four to six times a day. For most people, a fist represents somewhere between thirty and fifty grams of pure protein. To put this into perspective, for a bigger person, six to eight ounces of boneless, skinless chicken breast will yield approximately fifty grams of pure protein. A smaller person will need less protein per meal. Later, we will give you a precise formula so you can calculate the optimal amount of protein per day for your body.

If you combine a fist of lean, complete protein with a fist of slow-burning, low glycemic load carbohydrates such as vegetables or whole, fresh fruit, plus a small amount (about a thumb) of raw fat (such as raw nuts, raw seeds, avocado, Super Omega-3 caps, or olive oil), you will effectively keep your blood sugar rock solid for three to five hours.

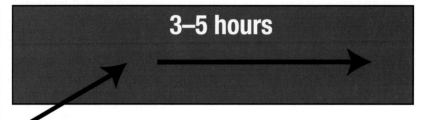

Consistently *stable blood sugar*

3–5 hours

Fist of lean protein+
Fist of slow-burning carbohydrates+
Thumb of essential fat or 1–2 capsules of Super Omega-3

And if you repeat this meal template (a fist + a fist + a thumb) four to six times a day, you will lose weight (fat), build muscle, and get lean. This meal template replicates the diet our ancestors thrived on for hundreds of thousands of years with literally no degenerative disease.

On the other hand, if you start your day with a glass of unsweetened orange juice (which is basically pure sugar) and combine that with a bowl of unsweetened breakfast cereal (also nearly pure sugar), a sliced banana and some nonfat milk, your blood sugar will spike, followed by an insulin spike, and you will store fat for the next eight to twelve hours. You will feel ravenously hungry all the time and crave sugar and other carbohydrates. You will feel sleepy and depressed and have a hard time concentrating. This is the kind of breakfast conventional wisdom and television ads promote, and it is a major reason why two-thirds of all Americans are overweight or obese and why Americans are some of the sickest people on earth.

Sleepiness after *any* meal is a classic sign that you are eating more carbohydrates than your body (and brain) can tolerate. Your body does not lie.

To optimize your body composition, you need to enhance your lean body mass (and it takes protein to build muscle) and burn body fat (you must keep your insulin from spiking if you ever hope to burn any fat).

What is the optimal amount of pure protein for your body? One hundred grams (3.5 ounces) of boneless, skinless chicken breast will yield twenty-five grams of *pure* protein. That means to get fifty grams of pure protein, a person would have to eat six to eight ounces of boneless, skinless chicken breast in one meal. If that sounds too complicated at first, there's a simple formula to calculate the optimal amount of protein for your body: You need at least one gram of pure protein per pound of body weight per day. For example, a two hundred–pound man would need approximately two hundred grams of pure protein per day spread out over four to six meals. Four to six meals may sound like a lot, but world-class athletes eat as many as ten to eleven meals a day. And they are in Olympic gold medal health. Also, some world-class athletes eat five hundred to six hundred grams of pure protein per day. Also for the record, their kidneys are perfect, but this is where maintaining optimal hydration becomes key.

Now, some of us (Sandy and me included) are especially carbohydrate sensitive or intolerant. Meaning we love carbs, but they don't love us. For those of us with metabolic dysfunctions, we have to eat about 50 percent more pure protein to keep our blood sugar stable. I am six feet, two inches tall and weigh 185 pounds. That means, according to our formula, I need approximately 185 grams of pure protein per day spread out over four to six meals. But I am very carbohydrate intolerant, so I need an additional 50 percent more pure protein to keep my insulin and my blood sugar under control. So that means I need about 185 grams of pure protein plus an additional 50 percent more (92.5 grams) for a total of approximately 277.5 grams of pure protein per day, which I round off to an even 300 grams of pure protein per day. I eat three hundred grams of pure protein spread out over six meals, or approximately fifty grams of pure protein per meal. This works for me. You may need more or less. Later, we'll help you figure out just how much you need.

How can you tell if you are carbohydrate intolerant, or if you have a dysfunctional metabolism? If you answer yes to one or more of the following questions, *your* body is telling you that you are eating more carbohydrates than your body can handle. Remember, we are all individuals. The key is to learn how to listen to *your* body. *Your* body does not lie.

1: **Do you have an ectomorphic body type?** Yes or no?

There are three basic body types: ectomorph, mesomorph, and endomorph. Ectomorphs have a linear body type. Mesomorphs are thick, stocky, and more muscular. Endomorphs are more round or pear shaped. There is a simple test to determine if you are ectomorphic, and if you are, how ectomorphic you are. Take your thumb and your middle finger (the longest finger) of your left hand, and wrap these two fingers around the smallest part of your right wrist. If your fingers touch or overlap, you have an ectomorphic body. The more your fingers overlap, the more ectomorphic you are. As an example, my thumb and middle finger overlap about an inch when I wrap them around the smallest part of my right wrist. I am very ectomorphic. Sandy's fingers overlap even more than mine do. We are both sugar sensitive. We both need more protein to keep our insulin from spiking and our blood sugar stable. By the way, having an ectomorphic body is not a bad thing. All the world's greatest endurance athletes (marathon runners, Ironman triathlon winners, and Olympic cross-country skiing champions) are all ectomorphs. We just have to eat more lean, complete protein and/or do more aerobic exercise to keep our insulin under control and our blood sugar stable.

2: Do you sometimes feel tired, depressed, sad, or feel sorry for yourself? Yes or no?

3: Do you find yourself often feeling hungry? Do you experience food cravings? Do you catch yourself obsessing about food? Yes or no?

4: Do you suffer from headaches, including migraines? Yes or no?

5: Do you suffer from PMS? If you're not sure, ask your partner or the people you work with. Yes or no?

6: Is your sleep ever disrupted? Do you ever wake up in the middle of the night or in the early hours just before dawn and can't get back to sleep? And as you are lying there, do you feel anxious, worried, or stressed about work or your personal life? Yes or no?

7: Do you ever experience anxiety or panic attacks? Do you ever feel overwhelmed? Yes or no?

8: Do you ever experience mood swings? Yes or no?

9: Do you ever experience fits of rage or uncontrolled anger where you "go off" on your spouse, children, or people you work with? Yes or no?

10: Do you have any excess body fat? Remember: Excess body fat for men is any body fat over 15 percent (the average American man is 26 percent body fat); excess body fat for women is any body fat over 22 percent (the average American woman is 36 percent body fat; the average American woman over fifty years of age is over 50 percent body fat). Yes or no?

If you answered yes to one or more of the above questions, it may be an indication that you are glucose intolerant and/or insulin resistant. If so, you may find that increasing your lean, complete protein intake and decreasing your carbohydrate intake just might make a positive difference in your struggle with excess weight, erratic moods, bouts of depression, or insomnia.

Exercise is essential to optimizing your body composition (building muscle and losing fat). The timing of your intake of protein is helpful if you want to maximize the benefits you get from your workouts. First and foremost, never exercise on an empty stomach. Why? Exercising on an empty stomach will burn off some of your precious muscle. The single most effective pre-workout meal you can put into your body first thing in the morning before your workout is half a protein shake. We will teach exactly how to make your pre-workout half-shake in the chapter on exercise.

Following your workout, there is a three-hour window (technically known as your anabolic window; anabolic means "to build"). To maximize the benefits you get from your workout, the most effective post-workout meal you can ingest immediately after your workout and *before* your shower is a full protein shake. Then, before your three-hour window closes, get in a second meal. Why? It is during your three-hour anabolic window that your body most efficiently and effectively absorbs both protein and carbohydrate, which further underscores the tremendous benefits of lean, complete protein at this time.

When should you eat your last meal of the day? A key to getting a sound night's sleep is stable blood sugar. Therefore, your last meal should be thirty to sixty minutes before you go to sleep. Never go to bed hungry. What do you eat just before you go to sleep? The template for your pre-sleep meal should sound familiar: a fist of lean, complete protein, a fist of slow-burning carbs, and a thumb of healthy fat. Please ignore the conventional wisdom about not eating after 6 or 7 PM. That bit of misinformation comes from the diet industry, which has a 98 percent failure rate. Try what we recommend and you will both sleep great and lose weight (fat). Listen to *your* body, not to the diet industry.

The following is a list of lean, complete proteins, in order, based on the biological value of protein.

- **100 percent whey protein isolate powder**.
- **Egg whites**.
- **Wild game** (venison, buffalo, antelope, moose, elk, ostrich, etc.).
- **Salmon, Ahi tuna**.
- **Turkey** (white meat, dark meat, no skin).
- **Fish** (of all kinds).
- **Tuna** (water packed only).
- **Chicken** (white meat only, no skin).
- **Shellfish** (lobster, crab, shrimp, oysters, mussels, clams).
- **Nonfat dairy**: nonfat milk, nonfat cheese, nonfat plain yogurt (no fruit on the bottom or sweeteners of any kind), nonfat or low-fat cottage cheese.

As with water, stock your house up with several kinds of lean protein and avoid running out. Remember, the cornerstone and the start of every one of your meals is a fist of lean, complete protein. Always eat your lean, complete protein first or with your meal. Avoid eating carbohydrates first or by themselves. Carbohydrates eaten first or by themselves will spike your insulin and then you will store fat for the next eight to twelve hours.

Chapter 10

Biological Essential: Essential Fat

Ninety-five percent of all Americans are omega-3 fat deficient.
—Udo Erasmus, PhD, *Fats that Heal, Fats that Kill,* 1993

If we go back to the very beginnings of life on earth, one of the fundamental requirements for any living organism was developing a way to separate the internal environment (what's inside the cell) from the external environment (what's outside the cell). Over time, deep in evolutionary history, primitive organisms struck on a solution: using fat to create a semi-permeable cell membrane. Today, all cell membranes are made out of molecules called phospholipids. Phospholipids are made from essential fats. Because the cell membranes of all living organisms are made from these special essential fats and goes back literally billions of years, essential fats are an integral part of our DNA, which programs the structure of every one of our cells.

Coming forward in time, from the beginnings of our modern species six to eight million years ago to today, essential fats have played a key role in what makes *Homo sapiens* unique. In the chapter on protein, we discussed how the invention of tools and our ancestors' ability to butcher carcasses dramatically improved the quality of our ancestors' diet. The consistent addition of meat from wild game, as well as bone marrow and brain, added not only high quality protein, but also significant amounts of essential fat. The muscles and organs of wild game animals are rich in omega-3 fat. Bone marrow and brain are an even richer source of omega-3 fat. From 2.6 million years ago until the arrival of *Homo sapiens* about two hundred thousand years ago, our ancestral brain roughly doubled in size. And we went from being bipedal apes to anatomically modern humans with the most advanced brain in history.

There are 2 essential fats: linoleic acid (omega-6) and alpha linolenic acid (omega-3). Biologic molecules are essential because our body has to have them but cannot synthesize them, therefore we have to ingest (eat) them. Essential fats are a critical component in the membranes of every single cell in our body. Essential fats allow our cell membranes to be flexible and fluid. In plain language, healthy cell membranes allow the good stuff like oxygen and nutrients to get into the cell, and the bad stuff like carbon dioxide to get out. The balance of omega-6 and omega-3 that we eat controls how permeable and flexible our cell membranes are. If we have a good ratio of (1:1) of omega-6 to omega-3, then all the cells in our body are healthy and fully functioning. But if our ratio gets out of balance due to a poor diet, and we take in more omega-6 than omega-3, then our cell membranes become less permeable and we become ill.

Since essential fats are crucially important to healthy cell membranes, they are crucial to the health of every organ in your body: your brain, your intestinal tract, your heart, your skin, and on and on. There are degrees of illness, but a deficiency or imbalance of essential fats can lead to conditions as minor as dry skin or as serious as suicidal depression and Alzheimer's.

Essential fat is *especially* crucial to brain development. Essential fats form the membranes of every neuron (a type of brain cell). And essential fats form the sheath that protects all the nerves in every part of our body. Research has shown that essential fat, especially omega-3, is critically important before conception, during the nine months the fetus spends in the womb, and the first eighteen months of life. Logically, that means essential fats are crucial for mothers-to-be, pregnant women, and lactating mothers. In fact, it is recommended that women thinking about becoming pregnant, pregnant women, and lactating mothers need 50 percent more essential fat, especially omega-3, than the rest of us. So during the developmental stage, both the baby and the mother need significant amounts of essential fat for optimal health and brain development. But the importance of essential fat in brain health does not stop at the developmental stage and the early years of growth. Lack of essential fats or an essential fat imbalance can lead to serious neurological problems and even mental illness throughout life.

Essential fats are also an integral component of our skin. The root cause of most skin problems is a lack of essential fats or an essential fat imbalance (too much omega-6). Examples include conditions such as eczema, acne, or psoriasis. But "skin" also has a broader meaning. As strange as this may sound, the inside of our lungs is really quite similar to the outside of our body. The inside of our lungs is actually a kind of skin. Lack of essential fats or an imbalance can lead to a whole range of respiratory problems, such as hay fever, allergies, bronchitis, sinusitis, and asthma. You don't need drugs to manage these health issues. You just need to change your diet.

The inside of our alimentary canal (our digestive tract) is also a kind of "skin." As a result, a lack of essential fats or an imbalance can lead to digestive issues, including acid reflux, ulcers, colitis, ileitis, or irritable bowel syndrome. You don't need drugs or surgery to manage these health issues. You simply need to change your diet. Your body doesn't lie.

And, of course, lack of essential fats or an imbalance (too much omega-6, which is the norm in America) can lead to the whole range of inflammation problems, including anything that ends in "itis," as well as heart and circulatory disease. Suffice it to say, it is impossible to be optimally healthy without a consistent and optimal intake of essential fat in a 1:1 ratio.

It turns out that the ancestral diet was naturally rich in omega-3 fat (Lindeberg 2010). As a result, people eating the ancestral diet had none of the degenerative diseases that plague modern man today. This ideal situation first began to change with the agricultural revolution, when the human diet began to shift from a diet high in wild meats that were rich in omega-3 fat to a cereal grain diet low in essential fat. And with this change came the first appearance of degenerative disease, which has now reached epidemic global proportions.

As part of our modern obesogenic environment, essential fats have either disappeared or have gotten dramatically out of balance. Around the year 1900, raw, healthy fats were still an integral part of the American diet. Over time, processed foods, including processed fats, became a bigger part of the American diet, gradually replacing fresh, natural foods. This trend of more and more highly processed foods accelerated after the

Second World War. And in the last thirty years, the vast majority of foods we find in our supermarkets are highly processed or totally synthetic. Shelf-life has become the driving commercial factor. Essential fats are, by nature, vulnerable to light, heat, and air. They spoil easily. By contrast, highly processed fats such as processed vegetable oils in clear bottles, partially hydrogenated fats in processed foods, and trans fats (the most toxic fats) are virtually indestructible with almost unlimited shelf life. As a result, omega-3 fat has almost disappeared from the American diet. In fact, 95 percent of all Americans are omega-3 fat deficient (Erasmus 1993). Omega-6 fat predominates.

Omega-6 fat is actually a biological double-edged sword. We do need some omega-6 fat, but the key is the *ratio* of our intake of omega-6 fat to omega-3 fat. The people who have the most ideal ratio of omega-6 to omega-3 fat are the Greenland Eskimos. The Greenland Eskimos have a ratio of 1:2.5 omega-6 to omega-3. Eskimos have the lowest level of inflammation of any people of earth. Because of their extremely low level of inflammation, Eskimos have virtually no degenerative disease. Remember, *the* root cause of all degenerative disease is inflammation. In contrast, the average American has a ratio of 20:1 or even 30:1 omega-6 to omega-3.

Like I said, omega-6 is, in fact, an essential fat. We do need some. But the ratio of omega-6 to omega-3 is critical because excess omega-6 gets converted to pro-inflammatory molecules. One of the fundamental reasons Americans have one of the highest levels of inflammation of any people on the face of the earth is our enormous intake of processed vegetable oils, which are all omega-6 fat. Processed vegetable oils, with corn oil being the worst, are an integral part of virtually all processed food and, of course, an integral component of fast-food. Our obesogenic environment aggressively promotes the massive intake of toxic fats.

So, essential fats play a mixed role in the Inflammation Challenge we talked about earlier. Omega-3 fat is clearly anti-inflammatory. Omega-6 fat in small amounts—never exceeding our omega-3 intake—is also anti-inflammatory. But if our intake of omega-6 gets out of balance and dominates our intake of omega-3 fats, we are in inflammatory trouble. The key is a balance of omega-6 to omega-3, with a ratio of 1:1 being optimal or maybe even a little more omega-3 than omega-6, like the Eskimos. But never the 20:1 or even 30:1 omega-6 to omega-3 ratios so common in our country today.

It should also be noted that hunter-gatherer societies did not suffer from any cognitive decline or degenerative diseases at all. They had no dementia, no senility, and no Alzheimer's whatsoever. They had no heart disease, diabetes, osteoporosis, or cancer. A major reason for this was their high, lifelong intake of omega-3 fat. And, of course, they did not eat any processed or toxic fats. This is an important lesson.

Essential fats come from foods that contain LA (linoleic acid/omega-6) or ALA (alpha linolenic acid/omega-3). The source most people think of first is salmon, particularly wild-caught salmon. And that is true. Essential fat is also found in some plants, particularly in raw flax seeds and raw flax seed oil. But essential fats are fragile, and omega-3 is five times more fragile than omega-6 (Erasmus 1993). This is a big reason why processed oils and fats with virtually unlimited shelf life have supplanted raw oils that are spoiled by light, heat, and/or exposure to air.

Also, unfortunately, our bodies are not very efficient at converting the essential fats to their more physiologically effective forms: EPA and DHA. Your body can only convert about 5 percent of the essential fat you eat into a form your body can really use. For example, three ounces of salmon contains 1.1 to 1.9 grams of omega-3 fat. If you ate a six-ounce portion (standard serving size) of salmon, you would take in between 2.2 and 3.8 grams of omega-3 fat. Five percent of 2.2 to 3.8 equals .11 to .19 grams of omega-3 fat your body can actually use. Optimal intake of omega-3 is somewhere between six grams and twelve grams per day. You would have to eat a lot of salmon to even get one day's worth of omega-3 fat! And to compound this problem, as we get older, our need for essential fats becomes even greater. Why? First, as we get older, inflammation becomes more of an issue. At any age, our bodies are not very efficient at converting the omega-3 fat found in natural foods like salmon or raw flax seeds into its more physiologically effective form EPA (eicosapentaenoic acid), or even more beneficial yet, DHA (docosahexaenoic acid). But as we get older, we become even less efficient. As a result, it is more effective for all of us, especially as we get older, to take DHA and EPA directly as a supplement. This is why molecularly distilled fish oil capsules are the most efficient and effective way to ensure that you get an optimal amount of omega-3 fat every day. And remember, molecularly distilled fish oil is even more important for pregnant women. It has been proven that an optimal intake of omega-3 fat can prevent both pre-term delivery and low birth weight babies and promote brain health. You can be even more efficient by taking additional DHA directly as a supplement, especially if you are focusing on brain development and/or battling depression.

Essential Fats and Weight Loss

When it comes to losing weight, omega-3 fat increases your body's oxidation rate. That means omega-3 fat will help your body burn more calories and more fat. Omega-3 fat increases metabolism. Omega-3 fat increases our energy level so we feel more like exercising and being active. Omega-3 fat increases our endurance so exercise feels easier and we feel like exercising longer. Omega-3 fat helps our kidneys dump excess water so we get rid of fluid retention. Omega-3 fat decreases cravings so it makes it easier for us to stay on our healthy eating plan.

The reason omega-3 fat eliminates our cravings for sugar and other carbohydrates is that omega-3 fat provides the real nutrition our body is looking for. Essential fat goes directly to our cells and tells our body that we have satisfied our real physiologic need so our appetite is turned down and our cravings subside. By including good sources of omega-3 fat like raw flax seed oil on our salads, we are able to keep our blood sugar more stable and avoid insulin spikes and fat storage. The more stable our blood sugar, the less hunger we experience. Remember, there is an inverse relationship between insulin and blood sugar. The higher your insulin spikes, the lower your blood sugar will crash. The lower your blood sugar, the more hunger you feel and the more intense your experience of hunger (Erasmus 1993).

The following is a list of the best sources of essential fats, in order, starting with the very best:

■ **Super Omega-3 Molecularly Distilled Fish Oil Capsules.** Most of us have heard that fish, especially fish like salmon, are healthy. That is true. However, there are at least three concerns with fish of any kind: mercury, PCBs, and dioxins. When fish is concentrated to get the oil, these three toxins are also concentrated. This is why it is so important to get molecularly distilled fish oil. Molecularly distilled fish oil is like distilled water. It's virtually 100 percent pure. No mercury, no PCBs, and no dioxins. Taking EPA and DHA directly is the most efficient and effective way to ensure your body receives its optimal amount of essential fat, so why not take the purest form available? We recommend that you take six to twelve capsules per day.

■ **Raw Organic Seeds.** At 58 percent, raw organic flax seeds contain the highest percentage of omega-3 fat. Our body cannot break down raw organic flax seeds. So to get the full benefit of this extraordinarily healthy food, we need to grind the seeds in a coffee grinder before adding them to our shake or salad. Other raw seeds include raw sunflower seeds, raw pumpkin seeds, and raw sesame seeds.

■ **Raw Organic Flax Seed Oil.** Raw organic flax seed oil has the greatest biological value of all the seed oils. Because heat damages or destroys essential fat, it is mandatory that raw organic flax seed oil be kept refrigerated both at the store and when you bring it home.

■ **Raw Nuts.** First, peanuts are not nuts. Peanut butter of any kind does not contain any essential fat at all. Peanut butter of any kind does not contain any usable protein. All peanut butter is junk food—despite all the marketing to the contrary. What we are looking for are tree nuts. Raw almonds are the most nutritious of all tree nuts. Other raw tree nuts include pecans, cashews, and walnuts.

■ **Raw Nut Butters.** If you enjoy the peanut butter experience— that is, the flavor and texture of peanut butter—we would suggest you try raw almond butter or raw cashew butter. These are both healthy foods that have a wonderful flavor and texture.

■ **Avocado.**

■ **Extra Virgin Olive Oil.** Any olive oil is good. Extra virgin olive oil comes from the first soft pressing and is considered the highest quality olive oil.

All the foods on this list are healthy. The one drawback is that all the foods on this list, except for the molecularly distilled fish oil capsules, are also very calorically dense. Along with its other benefits, this is one of the additional reasons we strongly suggest taking molecularly distilled fish oil capsules. Not only is molecularly distilled fish oil the purest and highest quality source of EPA and DHA, as well as the most easily absorbable form of omega-3, but it saves calories. Two capsules of molecularly distilled fish oil has about twenty-five calories. However, one pound of raw almonds, which is not much bigger than my fist, has 2,576 calories. You would have to do over five hours of nonstop aerobic exercise to burn off one pound of almonds. Even if you limit your intake of raw almonds to about ten to twelve nuts at a time (which is our recommended serving size), this contains about one hundred calories and only gives you a small fraction of the amount of EPA and DHA you receive from molecularly distilled fish oil capsules. And when it comes to avocadoes, they are 77 percent fat, so one pound of avocado has 752 calories. So, again, if you limit your intake of avocado to one small slice (about one-eighth of the fruit), you are fine, as this runs about one hundred calories—but again, you are receiving more calories and less EPA and DHA than you would otherwise obtain from molecularly distilled fish oil capsules. Keep all this in mind when deciding how much of your essential fat you choose to receive from molecularly distilled fish oil capsules and how much you ingest from whole food sources.

Remember, health is molecular. If we consistently give our body the molecules that we have evolved to thrive on, then we will be lean and healthy. Being lean and healthy is that simple. However, if we fall into the traps that conventional wisdom (marketing) sets for us, then we will be plagued by the full spectrum of degenerative diseases that plague modern man. Essential fats are two of those molecules.

Chapter 11

Biological Essential: Low Glycemic Load Carbohydrates

Ninety-nine percent of the pancreas is devoted to handling the digestion of fats and protein, while only 1 percent is devoted to handling sugar.
—David L. Williams, PhD, *Scientific Foundations of Biochemistry in Clinical Practice*, September 1994

Carbohydrate means sugar. If you keep that clearly in your mind, you are halfway to getting a good grip on carbohydrates and how to manage them. Of the three macronutrients (proteins, fats, and carbohydrates), carbohydrates are the least essential.

In fact, research has shown that Eskimos, before they were corrupted by modern society, ate a diet that was 98 percent protein and fat and only 2 percent carbohydrates. And yet they were some of the healthiest people on earth. Eskimos had the lowest level of inflammation of any people on earth, and as a result, they had none of the degenerative diseases caused by inflammation, such as heart disease, stroke, diabetes, etc. What may be even more ironic and enlightening is that Eskimos were eating over 2,000 mg of cholesterol every day (their diet consisted of six to eight pounds of raw meat per day), yet they had no heart disease whatsoever. That's right: They were eating seven times more cholesterol every single day of their lives than Americans, but they had zero heart disease. So much for the conventional wisdom that cholesterol causes heart disease. Or that a high-protein, high-fat diet causes heart disease (Lindeberg 2010). The body does not lie.

Let's look back into deep time and see what evolution has to tell us about the function of carbohydrates in human health and development. It turns out that the very earliest members of the human family tree were predominantly vegetarian. These were bipedal apes of the genus *Australopithecines*. As we trace our family tree forward in time from its deepest roots, we see a major split take place. *Australopithecines* become more specialized as vegetarians. Their front teeth get smaller and their back teeth, their cheek teeth or molars and pre-molars, get huge. *Australopithecines* developed huge chewing muscles, as revealed by a sagittal crest on the top of the skull where these powerful muscles attached. *Australopithecines* had small brains, not much larger than the brains of our nearest relative, the chimpanzee.

This branch culminated in *Australopithecus robustus*, affectionately known as the "nut cracker man" because his molars and chewing muscles were so huge. *Robustus'* molars were four times bigger than ours. He was a chewing machine. In fact, his teeth and chewing muscles approached those of a gorilla. Gorillas are 100 percent vegetarian. And despite over a million years of evolution, *Australopithecus robustus'* brain never got any bigger. The end result? *Australopithecus robustus* went extinct. *Australopithecus robustus* was too specialized, and when the climate changed, he could not adapt to the new environment. Darwinian survival is all about those organisms who are best adapted to a given environment. If you can't adapt, or if you get out-competed by an organism better adapted than you, you are history. That is the Darwinian reality of the world.

On the other branch of our ancestral tree, the genus *Homo* started with *Homo habilis*. (For the record, our evolutionary tree is much more complex than this, and there may have been as many as four or five different ancestral creatures all living at the same time in the same environment, but I don't want this to get too confusing.) *Homo habilis* invented tools, which *Australopithecines* never did. *Homo habilis* began to eat meat and omega-3 fat, which *Australopithecines* rarely did. *Homo habilis'* brain was 50 percent larger than that of the *Australopithecines*. This *Homo* branch of our evolutionary tree continued to grow larger and larger brains until we reached today's big-brained *Homo sapiens*. As the *Homo* brain grew, its digestive tract, from the teeth down through the gut, changed. The teeth got smaller and the gut got smaller and shorter (Aiello and Wheeler 1998).

The *Homo* branch became less gorilla-like. The *Homo* line became more generalized and, therefore, more adaptable. If you look at evolutionary history, those organisms that are the most generalized, and therefore the most adaptable, last the longest. Examples of generalist organisms that are highly adaptable include rats, cockroaches, and *Homo sapiens*. Those organisms that are very specialized and require a very specific niche are the most vulnerable to change. Examples include koalas, pandas, and gorillas, all of which are on the brink of extinction.

The *Homo* branch got into a feed-forward loop starting with the invention of tools, which allowed early *Homo* to butcher carcasses deserted by predators. Tools allowed the genus *Homo* access to highly nutritious food (wild game meat, marrow, and brain). Highly nutritious food enhanced brain growth. A bigger, smarter brain enabled the genus *Homo* to evolve from an opportunistic scavenger to a highly skilled hunter with more and more lethal weapons at his disposal. The supply of nutritious meat increased dramatically. By the time *Homo sapiens* arrived on the scene about two hundred thousand years ago, there were no animals that we couldn't kill and eat. And by approximately one hundred thousand years ago, when *Homo sapiens* left Africa, we were able to adapt to every environment on the earth, from equatorial Africa to northern Siberia. We lived on everything from antelopes we killed on the African savanna to reindeer herds and wooly mammoths during the Ice Age. The point I'm trying to make is that *the key* to our evolution from our primitive ancestors to the most dominant species on the planet today was meat (lean, complete protein) and fat (especially omega-3 fat). Carbohydrates were a distant third.

The roots of our present-day global obesity epidemic began ten to twelve thousand years ago with the advent of the agricultural revolution. That was the moment in human history when a major shift began to take place in the human diet. The major shift was from a meat- and fat-based diet (wild game) on which we had thrived for millions of years to a sugar-based diet based on cereal grains.

Too many carbohydrates cause big problems, both short- and long-term, for a mother and her developing fetus. As this baby matures, he/she is two to four times more likely to be overweight, diabetic, and have heart disease or stroke later in life.

A common practice in our culture is to give our babies and toddlers a juice bottle (virtually 100 percent sugar) on a regular basis to keep them quiet. When this is done, the growing baby will likely get fat and be an overweight child, not to mention having a mouth full of cavities. Later in life, this may lead to that child becoming an obese adult who suffers from gum disease (gingivitis) and/or periodontal disease. Both of these situations predispose that individual to heart disease later. And all of these are a direct result of over-carbing. Pregnant mothers, lactating mothers, and growing children need 50 percent more lean, complete protein and 50 percent more essential omega-3 fat. The last thing they need is too many carbohydrates.

But given our modern obesogenic environment, most Americans are encouraged, almost pressured, to overeat and overdrink carbohydrates. The first place to look is the Food Pyramid, which has now been updated as The Plate. In either case, the USDA (the United States Department of Agriculture) is teaching and encouraging Americans to eat a diet that is approximately 75 percent sugar. Remember: *All* carbohydrates are sugar.

How did this destructive way of eating evolve? Early in recorded history, pure sugar was very expensive and hard to get. But beginning at the end of the Second World War, and especially in the last thirty years, simple and refined sugars (carbohydrates) became cheaper and much easier to get than healthier foods. Sugar is also highly addictive, since sugar acts on the reward center in our brain just like addictive drugs do.

As food manufacturers and advertisers began to understand how addictive these foods were, they knew they had tapped into a market that would always demand their products. This presented an unbelievable opportunity for them. By manufacturing high-sugar, low-cost foods, they too were now "addicted" to sugar (albeit it in a different way). As a result, 90 percent of all Americans spend their entire lives addicted to sugar.

The tangible results are highly visible. Sixty-seven percent of all Americans are overweight. One-third of all adult Americans are medically obese. The technical definition of medical obesity is anyone who is thirty or more pounds above their ideal weight. A good rule of thumb for a person's ideal healthy weight is what you weighed in high school, provided you were not already overweight at that time. Optimally, you should weigh what you weighed when you graduated from high school or less—your whole life.

As one result of this encouragement (e.g., advertising, particularly TV advertising, combined with cheap sugar and sugary drinks), Americans ingest more sugar per capita than any other people on earth. According to the United States Department of Agriculture, the per capita consumption of sugar is 156 pounds per year for every man, woman, and child in the country. That's thirty-one five-pound bags of sugar per year for every single American. The biggest single increase over the last twenty years has been in the area of sweetened drinks, including sweetened teas, sports drinks, and fruit drinks. Sugar shows up in the obvious places like cakes and cookies. But sugar also shows up in places like ketchup, yogurt, and peanut butter. And many people have the misguided notion that fat-free means calorie free. When manufacturers remove fat, which gives food so much flavor, they frequently compensate by increasing the sugar content. Most fat-free foods and salad dressings are nearly pure sugar.

America is suffering from an epidemic of metabolic disorders or dysfunctions, including glucose intolerance, insulin resistance, and diabetes. According to the 2011 National Diabetes Fact Sheet (released on January 26, 2011) by the American Diabetes Association, 25.8 million children and adults in the United States—8.3 percent of the population—have diabetes: 18.8 million people are diagnosed; 7.0 million people are undiagnosed; and 79 million people are pre-diabetic.

Of all diabetics, over 90 percent are type 2. Type 2 diabetes is 100 percent preventable and 100 percent manageable without drugs. However, let's look at what our environment (the American Diabetes Association) teaches us in terms of how to manage diabetes. Keep in mind, diabetes is when the person's body has a problem handling carbohydrates (sugar). With diabetes, the person's body does *not* have a problem with protein or fat. Their body just has a problem with sugar (carbohydrates).

Let's look at the new (2011) Diabetes Plate. The changes from the Food Pyramid and the new Plate to the Diabetes Plate turn out to be confusing and not much of an improvement. The new Diabetes Plate instructs you to take your plate and divide it in half, then fill half your plate with up to 1 cup cooked vegetables or up to 2 cups raw vegetables. Either of these choices will give you about 10–15 grams of carbohydrates. So far, so good. But then the ADA tells us to fill one-quarter of our plate with three-quarters to 1 cup of starchy food like beans. This will add between fifteen and thirty grams of *additional* carbs. Then we are told to fill the last quarter of our plate with protein. This can be meat (no additional carbs) or tofu. One hundred grams of tofu (about 3.5 ounces) will only provide about seven grams of protein (woefully short of the thirty to fifty grams per meal needed by most people) and an additional two to five grams of carbs. Then we are told to drink an eight-ounce glass of nonfat or low-fat milk. Either kind of milk will add twelve more grams of carbs (lactose) to our meal. Assuming that the protein chosen is 3.5 ounces of boneless, skinless chicken breast, which provides twenty-five grams of protein, this suggested meal is approximately 50 to 60 percent carbohydrates with very little protein or fat to slow its absorption. And this is assuming that our diabetic adheres to the very strict portion guidelines set out by the new Plate.

The American Diabetes Association offers "Breakfast on the Go" suggestions. One suggestion is a recipe for Banana Ginger Muffins. They are made with flour, unsweetened applesauce, brown sugar, and 2 mashed bananas. Each muffin contains 28 grams of carbs, 3 grams of fat, and 5 grams of protein. That means each muffin is 72 percent carbs (sugar), 16 percent fat, and 12 percent protein. Then we are told to top our muffins with "fresh berries and a dollop of fresh yogurt." For someone with a proven metabolic disorder (diabetes), a breakfast like this is courting disaster.

As a final comment on the new and improved American Diabetes Plate, they present a list of super foods for diabetics. At the top of their list are beans. Beans are one of the highest glycemic load carbohydrates. High glycemic load carbohydrates raise insulin the most, and therefore cause the most problems for a person whose metabolism is glucose intolerant and/or insulin resistant. Also on their list of super foods for diabetics are whole grains and whole grain products. If you simply look at a chart of high glycemic load carbohydrates and/or read Lindeberg's book, *Food and Western Disease* (2010), it becomes starkly clear that the new American Diabetes Plate is grossly out of sync with current scientific research.

This is the environment we live in. The organizations with the responsibility to help decrease and manage the diabetes epidemic in this country are offering suggestions that are guaranteed to turn the majority of even healthy people into diabetics. You can begin to see why our environment is obesogenic. With cheap sugar and sugary drinks everywhere you turn, combined with the standard Food Pyramid/Plate, which is approximately

75 percent sugar, and the new Diabetes Plate, which is still a high-sugar diet, the American people are understandably lost and confused.

As we get older, our bodies become less adaptable to changes and less tolerant of insults. We become less glucose tolerant and more insulin resistant. Nothing ages the human body faster than sugar in all its forms. So just when we are least able to tolerate it, many of the problems associated with sugar kick in. We have a harder time keeping our blood sugar stable. The more unstable our blood sugar, the faster we age and the more glucose intolerant we become. It becomes a vicious cycle.

As we get older, it becomes more challenging to keep our weight and our body fat under control. Excess body fat accelerates the aging process and contributes to glucose intolerance and insulin resistance. Again, the vicious cycle is perpetuated. And yet, as we look at how hunter-gatherers aged, the picture is very different than what we see today. Hunter-gatherer people had no obesity, cognitive issues, or degenerative disease. Hunter-gatherers ate no refined sugar, flour, grains, beans, dairy, or alcohol. If you want to age successfully, the hunter-gatherer model of eating is the best blueprint of optimal human health you will find.

In the Aging Challenge, we identified inflammation as a major factor in aging today. However, even older hunter-gatherers had no inflammation. If we compare our diet to the hunter-gatherer diet, the differences may be illuminating. There are several causes of chronic inflammation, including excess body fat. Remember, excess body fat for men is any body fat over 15 percent, and excess body fat for women is any body fat over 22 percent. Simple and refined carbohydrates are the single biggest causes of excess body fat. In fact, excess body fat is proof positive that the person is eating more carbohydrates than their body can tolerate. Simple and refined carbohydrates raise insulin. Any time a person over-carbs (eats too many carbohydrates in a sitting) and/or eats carbohydrates of any kind on an empty stomach, they will trigger a blood sugar spike followed by an insulin spike.

Insulin is a hormone that your pancreas secretes as part of homeostasis. Homeostasis is your body's mechanism to keep your internal environment as stable as it can. Your body attempts to keep all its parameters within optimal ranges. When any biomarker goes above or below its optimal range, your body swings into action to correct the situation. When blood sugar spikes, your pancreas responds by secreting insulin. The job of insulin is to take the excess glucose out of your bloodstream by converting it to either glycogen, if your muscle or liver stores of glycogen are at less than optimal levels, or to triglycerides, which are then stored in your fat cells. (If you have high triglycerides, *the* cause is too many carbohydrates.)

Insulin is *the* most powerful fat storing hormone in your body. But if your body is insulin resistant, then your pancreas has to secrete more and more insulin to drive the excess blood sugar into your fat cells. Chronically elevated levels of insulin are a major cause of inflammation. To compound the problem, if your pancreas over-releases insulin and drives your blood sugar too low, this is a major stress event. Your brain has to have glucose. Your body exists to keep your brain alive. Any time your blood sugar crashes, your adrenal glands come to the rescue. Your adrenal glands release cortisol, the most powerful stress hormone in your body. Cortisol immediately begins to convert some of your muscle (your precious lean body mass) into glucose (because muscle is easy to convert to glucose) to bring your blood sugar back up to keep your brain alive. Excess cortisol facilitates fat storage (makes you fatter) and raises inflammation levels.

So now we have a vicious cycle of three of the major causes of inflammation in a feed-forward cycle. And the entire inflammation cascade was precipitated by either over-carbing and/or eating carbohydrates on an empty stomach (like drinking a glass of orange juice first thing in the morning).

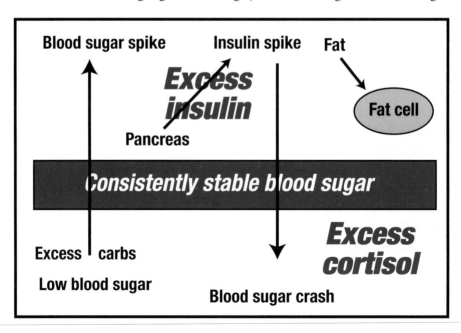

The above scenario takes place in most people's bodies several times a day. You can see why Americans have the highest inflammation levels in the world. We experience a never-ending cycle of excess sugar/carbohydrates, glucose spikes, insulin spikes, fat storage, blood sugar crashes, and cortisol surges. This is all encouraged by our environment and conventional wisdom. Most people are trapped in the downward spiral of sugar addiction and its consequences, including inflammation and degenerative disease. Hunter-gatherers were lean, got lots of exercise so they had no insulin resistance, and never binged on refined carbohydrates because none existed.

Carbohydrates come in several different forms, but the thing to always remember is this: Carbohydrates, no matter what form you find them in, are always sugar. Carbohydrates are never protein or fat. Carbohydrates can only be sugar. You may hear discussions about simple carbohydrates versus complex carbohydrates in the media and get the impression that complex carbohydrates are healthy and simple carbohydrates are unhealthy. Any time you eat more carbohydrates than your body can handle, regardless of the kind, you are in trouble. It all comes down to insulin. If carbohydrates drive your insulin up, you are in trouble. Later, we will teach you a simple and direct way you can measure your body's response to carbohydrates in the "Listen to YOUR Body" chapter.

There are two common ways to measure how fast carbohydrates convert to glucose and how much they raise your insulin. One measure is called the glycemic index (GI). Comparing carbohydrates to glucose with a score of one hundred (or a slice of white bread, which is also one hundred) carbohydrates are given a score. The closer the score is to one hundred, the faster the carbohydrate breaks down and converts to glucose. If the score is over one hundred, then obviously the carbohydrate converts to glucose very rapidly. The problem is that some carbohydrates do not break down as fast, but ultimately raise your insulin levels to very unhealthy levels none the less. So a new index was devised at Harvard Medical School. This index is called the glycemic load index (GLI). The GLI takes the GI score and multiplies it by the grams of carbohydrate per serving. This score gives a much more accurate depiction of the amount a given carbohydrate ultimately raises your insulin.

Some surprises showed up with the GLI. Some carbohydrates that scored low on the GI scored the highest on the GLI. For example, beans are considered a low GI carbohydrate. But both beans and grains contain a high number of grams of carbohydrate, making them actually a high glycemic *load* carbohydrate. So ultimately beans (and legumes of any kind) and grains raise insulin significantly, and as a result, are fattening and inflammatory.

Other carbohydrates don't show up because they are metabolized differently. Fructose is a good example. Fructose is often recommended as a healthy sugar. In fact, fructose is one of the worst carbohydrates. Why? Fructose is metabolized by your liver, rather than by your small intestine. When fructose enters your liver, it is converted into triglycerides (blood fats), rather than showing up as blood glucose. Normally, when a carbohydrate is ingested, blood sugar (glucose) rises, and this stimulates the pancreas to release insulin. Any excess glucose that is not needed is then converted into triglycerides (blood fats) by insulin, and then those triglycerides (fats) are stored in your fat cells. Because fructose bypasses that pathway, people who promote fructose are giving you the false impression that fructose is healthy. Excessive use of fructose will make you fat and is detrimental to your health. Excessive use of fructose will actually produce a fatty liver, just as if the person had been an alcoholic. With the rampant use of high fructose corn syrup, this is becoming a common condition.

Alcohol is another carbohydrate, like fructose, that is metabolized by your liver. This is how alcohol manufacturers can get away with advertising that such and such an alcohol has zero net carbs. This is just a technicality and another way food manufacturers are playing word games with you. Alcohol is distilled sugar. If we look at the label of alcohol, we see there is no fat, no protein, and *apparently* no carbs. But there are, in fact, *calories* in alcohol. So what exactly are the calories in alcohol made of? Because alcohol is metabolized by your liver, instead of the small intestine, the alcohol manufacturers can legally say zero net carbs. In fact, nothing will raise your triglycerides faster than alcohol.

In our obesogenic society, it is caveat emptor (let the buyer beware), meaning you are on your own to negotiate the deceptive labyrinth created by food manufacturers. If you want to know the real carbohydrate content of any food, subtract the total calories that come from protein and the total calories from fat from the total calories per serving. One hundred percent of the calories that are left are carbohydrates (sugar).

Other forms of carbohydrate/sugar that are used to mislead the public are sugar alcohols such as xylitol, sorbitol, mannitol, HSH, and glycerol.

Again, by playing semantic games, food manufacturers are permitted to omit sugar alcohols as a source of carbohydrates (sugar). This is because sugar alcohols are only *partially* digested in our small intestine. But because they are only partially digested, they commonly cause abdominal pain, bloating, gas, and diarrhea and can also be converted to triglycerides and stored as fat in our fat cells, making us fatter.

In addition to low-calorie sugar alcohols, food manufacturers have invented artificial sweeteners and artificially sweetened diet sodas that do not contain any calories at all. Zero calories! A dieter's dream come true, right? Well, maybe, but not so fast.

There have actually been a number of studies done on diet sodas and artificial sweeteners. A major ten-year study was done by Sharon P. Fowler and a team of doctors at the University of Texas Medical School. The study compared people who drank regular soda with people who drank diet soda. The study compared the risk of becoming overweight or obese. All the participants were of normal weight at the start of the ten-year study. Surprisingly, the study found that nearly all of the obesity risk came from diet sodas. In fact, there was a 41 percent risk of becoming overweight for every can or bottle of diet soft drink the person consumed each day.

For diet soft-drink drinkers, the risk of becoming overweight or obese was (Fowler 2005):

36.5 percent for up to a half-can each day
37.5 percent for one-half to one can each day
54.5 percent for one to two cans each day
57.1 percent for more than two cans each day

A study on aging just published in 2011 by a team of epidemiologists at the University of Texas Medical Center at San Antonio, including Helen P. Hazuda, PhD, showed that diet sodas increased waist circumference in humans. The San Antonio Longitudinal Study of Aging did an enrollment exam and three follow-up exams over a ten-year period. The results: Diet soft drink users as a group experienced 70 percent greater increases in waist circumference compared with non-users. Frequent users, defined as those people who consumed two or more diet sodas per day, experienced waist circumference increases 500 percent greater than non-users (Hazuda et al 2011). Dr. Hazuda summed up diet sodas with this comment: "They may be free of calories, but they are *not* free of consequences," and abdominal fat is the worst kind of fat.

In animals, Ganesh Halade, PhD, and Gabriel Fernandes, PhD, showed that aspartame (Equal), an artificial sweetener used in diet sodas and other products, raised both glucose and insulin levels and encouraged the development of diabetes (Halade and Fernandes 2011).

The above studies make it clear that by interacting with your body's sense of satisfaction, the chemicals in artificial sweeteners confuse your brain's natural satiety hormones. Artificial sweeteners used in literally thousands of products, including diet sodas, cereals, desserts, and a whole range of so-called "sugar-free" products, thereby make you crave more sugar and sweet foods, which contributes to the epidemic of obesity and metabolic disorders.

The moral of the artificial sweetener story is simple: Just because the label on a product says "sugar free" or "calorie free" or "diet" does not mean that the product will actually help you lose weight. In fact, artificially sweetened foods and drinks are some of the most fattening, most powerful appetite stimulating foods you can eat. If you are trying to lose weight, it does not make sense to be eating or drinking appetite stimulants. Artificial sweeteners are yet another prime example of the Black Box of Conventional Wisdom (marketing) designed to deceive unsuspecting people into believing you can get something for nothing. In life, there are *no* free lunches. *Your* body does not lie.

Be sure to look below the surface to make sure you are getting the full story on what you are about to eat and the effect of that food on your body fat and your health. Sugar comes in a lot of different forms. And many people do not recognize sugar in all its different guises. The obvious sugars are the hardcore sugars: cakes, pies, cookies, candy, ice cream, soda, etc. But many people do not realize that *all* flour products are nearly pure sugar and will definitely make you fat. Examples of flour products include: breads of any kind, pasta of any kind, bagels, pancakes, waffles, chips of any kind, and all the ready-to-eat-cereals that take up an entire aisle in your grocery store. They are all virtually pure sugar.

Here is a simple example to prove the point. One cup of plain Shredded Wheat (49 grams, which is only 1.75 ounces of cereal) has 167 calories. Five calories are from fat, the label says. So 167 minus five equals 162 calories. There are five grams of protein, the label says. A gram of protein contains four calories. So five grams of protein times four calories per gram equals twenty calories of protein: 162 minus 20 leaves 142 calories. We have eliminated the protein and fat, so all that is left is sugar (carbohydrates). One hundred forty-two divided by four (one gram of carbohydrate contains four calories) equals 35.5 grams of carbohydrate; 35.5 grams of sugar equals 8.9 teaspoons of sugar in one cup (1.75 ounces) of plain Shredded Wheat. Thirty-five grams of sugar, or almost nine teaspoons of sugar, is almost exactly what you get in a standard Snickers bar.

Another way of looking at this cereal, plain Shredded Wheat, is to take the total number of carbohydrate calories (142 per 1.75 ounce serving) and divide that by the total calories (per 1.75 ounce serving). When we divide 142 by 162 we discover that literally 88 percent of all the calories in plain Shredded Wheat are sugar. It's just a candy bar in sheep's clothing. And let's be honest with ourselves here. Most people will have more like two cups, so that would mean you need to double all of these amounts. Therefore, the average person is basically having two candy bars for breakfast.

For all practical purposes, the vast majority of all the calories in all flour products is sugar. To drive this point home, Dr. Walter Willett, MD, PhD, wrote: "When you eat a piece of whole wheat bread, by the time it hits your stomach, you've got sugar water." That is how fast flour turns to sugar.

In reality, there is no such thing as whole grain bread. If it was truly whole grain, you would have a pile of wheat. Once you grind wheat into wheat flour, you have predigested it. Grinding wheat into flour does what your body's digestive system would do over a period of hours. It is a fact of physics: The greater the surface area, the faster something dissolves. The smaller the particle, the greater the surface area. When you grind wheat berries into flour, you have reduced the wheat to tiny particles. In the process, you have exponentially increased the surface area. Hence Dr. Willett's quote.

When you eat a piece of so-called whole wheat bread, the flour converts into simple sugar so fast that the simple sugar enters your bloodstream through the capillaries in your mouth. All breads are made out of flour. Again, in reality, there is no such thing as "flourless" bread. The term "flourless" just means that the flour is ground a little more coarsely than pastry flour. The difference is cosmetic and semantic—and misleading. So-called "flourless" bread will spike your blood sugar, spike your insulin, and make you fat.

One of the most popular formats for a meal in this country is a sandwich. Think of a sandwich as two pieces of chocolate cake with whatever you put between them. You're never going to get lean eating sandwiches.

The lesson: When you look at the Nutrition Facts on a carbohydrate source like a box of cereal, the only thing you are concerned about is the total number of carbohydrates. The rest of the numbers are just games the food manufacturer is playing with you to try to convince you that a box of highly processed sugar is somehow a healthy food. There were no boxes of cereal one hundred thousand years ago.

What do carbohydrates have to do with losing weight? The single most important concept when it comes to losing weight is insulin management. Why? Because insulin is *the* hormone that makes us fat.

Insulin is a classic two-edged sword: It cuts both ways. We have to have insulin to live. But out-of-control insulin wreaks havoc in your body. Insulin converts sugar (glucose) into triglycerides (blood fats) and then stores those triglycerides (fats) in your fat cells. Insulin also prevents the burning of any body fat. Whenever insulin is elevated, it trumps all other hormones when it comes to fat storage. When insulin is elevated, insulin creates a one-way gate into your fat cells. Insulin will only put fat *in* to your fat cells. Insulin will *not* let any fat *out* of your fat cells. Think of those grates you drive over when you return a rental car. The sign says that backing up will result in severe tire damage. Insulin is that powerful.

If insulin is the key, then the next question becomes, "What raises insulin?" And the answer is carbohydrates (sugar in any form). This is why eating carbohydrates by themselves is a blood sugar disaster. Carbohydrates of any kind on an empty stomach will immediately spike your blood sugar, which will immediately spike your insulin.

Let me share with you a real life example. As I mentioned, I have been personally coaching people since 1979. Many of my clients have been diabetics. Whenever I work with a diabetic, I insist that they take their blood glucose levels six times a day and write it down. I had one client who had been an insulin-dependent type 2 diabetic for seventeen years. He lived in a two-story house. He got up one morning, walked downstairs to his kitchen, and ate three grapes. He suddenly realized he had not tested his blood glucose yet that morning. He quickly went back upstairs, pricked his finger, and tested his blood glucose level. Optimal fasting blood glucose levels are 70 to 85. When my client took his blood glucose level after eating just three grapes, it was already over 300. Long story short, within sixty days, I helped my client get off all his drugs, and he has been able to manage his blood sugar with nutrition and exercise ever since.

If you spike your insulin, it will stay elevated for hours, and you will prevent any fat from being released from your fat cells and burned. A blood sugar spike followed by an insulin spike will result whenever we eat too many carbohydrates in a given meal, such as a plate of pasta. So the number one key to managing insulin is to avoid eating carbohydrates of any kind on an empty stomach or eating too many carbohydrates in a given meal. Most people can only handle about fifteen to twenty-five grams of carbs in a given meal. Now you can appreciate even more the absurdity of the American Diabetes Association recommending breakfast muffins that are 72 percent carbs, for a diabetic no less. We will teach you in the chapter, "Listen to YOUR Body" exactly how to monitor your body so you can dial in the optimal carbohydrate intake for your body (Holt 1996).

Lean, complete protein also raises insulin. But insulin's response to protein is very different than insulin's response to carbohydrates (sugar). First and foremost, protein does *not* spike blood sugar. So you never get an insulin spike from protein. Protein causes a very slow and gradual rise in blood sugar over several hours. Second, lean, complete protein triggers the release of a hormone called glucagon that counters the actions of insulin. Glucagon raises our blood sugar slowly over time to allow for the absorption of amino acids into our liver, where they are converted to glucose. From an evolutionary biology point of view, this makes complete sense. Glucagon makes *Homo sapiens* much more of a best-surviving generalist. If all our ancestor had to eat one hundred thousand years ago was a big chunk of mammoth meat, he could still make the glucose required by his brain. For example, if you were to eat nothing but one medium-sized boneless, skinless chicken breast for a meal, about 25 percent of that chicken breast would end up as glucose to keep your brain happy.

Fat does not cause the release of insulin. That is why we recommend that you include some healthy fat with each of your meals. Healthy fat, along with lean, complete protein, dramatically slows the release of carbohydrates into your bloodstream, so your blood sugar never spikes, and therefore your insulin never spikes, and you never store fat.

The key is to discover the right balance of lean proteins, healthy fats, and slow-burning carbohydrates for *your* body. We will talk more about how to achieve the optimal balance for your body in the last section of this book, "Effective Actions."

The following list of carbohydrates is prioritized based upon which carbohydrates raise your insulin the least. To maximize fat loss, stick with the first two or three categories until you reach your ideal body weight: leafy green vegetables and vegetables. Use fruit sparingly. Make sure you include a generous fist of lean, complete protein and some healthy fat with each of your meals.

Carbohydrate List:

- **Leafy green vegetables** (unlimited). Leafy green vegetables are your first choice. Why? Leafy green vegetables contain the fewest carbohydrates and the greatest amount of nutritional value. Leafy green vegetables are the most nutrient-dense of all the carbohydrates. Leafy green vegetables break down the slowest. Leafy green vegetables raise your insulin the least. Leafy green vegetables are high in vitamins, minerals, and antioxidants. You can eat unlimited amounts of leafy green vegetables. Variety is important. Greener is better. Organic is better. Examples include: arugula, bok choy, chard, endive, escarole, romaine, spinach, and watercress. There are dozens more leafy green vegetables.

- **Vegetables** (fresh or frozen, not canned: up to two cups per meal). Examples include: Brussels sprouts, cabbage, cauliflower, celery, bell peppers, squash, tomatoes, zucchini, green beans, okra, asparagus, onions, leeks, carrots, jicama, radishes, and water chestnuts.

- **Whole, fresh fruit or frozen, unsweetened fruit** (up to one cup per meal). Fruit, in general, has a much higher carbohydrate content than vegetables, so you need to limit your intake to no more than one medium piece of fruit (like one medium apple) or one cup of fresh or frozen, unsweetened fruit. Examples include: apples, oranges, pears, peaches, apricots, and figs. Berries are the best fruits for losing weight because they break down the slowest. Why? Three things slow down the assimilation of glucose: protein, fat, and fiber. Berries contain lots of seeds. Seeds are fiber. So some of the most desirable fruits in terms of health, stable blood sugar, and losing weight are blackberries, boysenberries, and blueberries, with strawberries being the best of all. If you are going to use fruit as part of a meal, choose berries first as they will raise your insulin the least.

- **Yams or sweet potatoes** (one-half cup ideally, but no more than one cup cooked with each meal). Yams and sweet potatoes are still healthy carbohydrates, but as we move down our list, these foods raise your insulin levels much more than previously listed vegetables or even fruit. Use cautiously.

- **Beans, peas, lentils** (one-half cup cooked with each meal). As with yams and sweet potatoes, use legumes cautiously.

- **Whole grains** (one-half cup cooked with each meal). First of all, whole grains means whole. What do we mean by whole? Whole means no "whole grain products," which are a hoax. It also means no pre-prepared grains. No instant rice. Examples of acceptable whole grains include: wild rice, brown rice (both long grain and short grain), corn, wheat, rye, barley, and oat groats. You may be puzzled by the last several names. All these cereal grains cook at the same speed and the same way as brown rice. In fact, you can cook them in your rice cooker, if you have one. However, whole grains have a fairly high glycemic load, so use sparingly.

Important note: You are to have only *one* of the carbohydrates from the lists above with each of your meals, not one from *each* list. For breakfast, for example, you may choose up to one cup of fruit with your lean protein and essential fat. For lunch, you may choose a big salad of leafy greens with your lean protein and essential fat. For dinner, you may choose two cups of vegetables with your lean protein and essential fat. You may also combine different carbohydrates from each group, provided you do not go over the allotted amount. For example, you may choose a half-cup of fruit combined with one cup of vegetables.

Now you have learned that we have to have protein (the eight essential amino acids) if we want to be healthy and lean. We have to have fat (especially omega-3). It is ironic that the one macronutrient, carbohydrates, we need the least of, and the macronutrient that is the least essential for health, is the one promoted by conventional wisdom to be 60–75 percent of our total caloric intake. In fact, you can actually live on meat and fat alone. Eskimos have been doing this for tens of thousands of years.

The only exceptions are endurance athletes. One of the biggest challenges for endurance athletes of any kind (e.g., marathoners, bikers, triathletes, swimmers, cross-country skiers) is replacing their glycogen stores in their liver and in their muscles. Glycogen is the stored form of glucose. When a marathoner runs out of glycogen, he bonks. He goes from running to the survival shuffle. His race is over. He has to drag himself across the finish line. The name of the game in a marathon or any kind of distance endurance event is to get the other guy to go anaerobic.

In anaerobic metabolism, all we can burn are sugar and muscle. Once we go anaerobic, we are going to burn through our limited supply of glycogen very quickly. World-class marathoner runners have trained their bodies to burn fat very efficiently. So efficiently, in fact, that they can burn fat while running at a 4:40-minute-mile pace for the entire marathon. They never bonk or hit the wall.

Unfortunately, the popular media picks up on all this advice to elite endurance athletes about carbohydrate loading. Maybe you've seen a video of some world-class athlete putting away massive amounts of carbs, and yet he is 4–5 percent body fat. The general public and/or weekend warrior athletes think they can eat the same way a world-class athlete eats, despite the fact that the athlete is running over one hundred miles every week or biking hundreds of miles a week in training. As a result, these weekend warrior athletes are over-carbing and slugging down performance drinks, and all they end up doing is getting fat.

All the nutritional advice you hear for athletes is really for that top 1 percent who are training seriously. The rest of us—and this is the unfortunate truth—have to severely curtail our carb intake or our insulin will spike and we will store fat. If you have any doubt which category you fall into (the upper 1 percent of all endurance athletes or the other 99 percent of us mere mortals) just take all of your clothes off and stand naked in front of a full-length mirror. If you don't have six-pack abs, you are in the other 99 percent with the rest of us.

Your body does not lie.

Fortunately, the good news is that if you follow our program, you might not end up a world-class athlete, but you just might look like one.

Chapter 12

Biological Essential: Full Body Aerobic Exercise

*When you finish a good workout, you don't simply feel better.
You feel better about yourself.*
—George Allen, football coach

Evolutionary biology is about how our biology has evolved over time. Somewhere in the neighborhood of six to eight million years ago, we split off from a common ancestor that we shared with chimpanzees. Our common ancestor lived primarily in trees, and when it did move around on the ground, it probably knuckle-walked, the way chimpanzees still do.

The most important criterion that separates our direct ancestors from the other species on our evolutionary family tree is bipedalism. From the very beginning, we walked upright on two legs. From the very start, we were good walkers. But over time, our bodies evolved so we became exceptional walkers. Our hunter-gatherer ancestors walked miles and miles every single day of their lives, hunting wild game and foraging. Hunter-gatherers often walked fifteen to twenty miles a day. The lesson? Walking and being physically active is an integral part of what it means to be a human being, a *Homo sapien*. Activity and vigorous exercise are a Biological Essential if we want to be lean and optimally healthy. You can get thin without exercise, but you can't get lean. Thin is weak. Lean is strong and fit.

Unfortunately, our modern, obesogenic environment does not encourage exercise. We have become a sedentary nation. In fact, epidemiologists at Atlanta's Centers for Disease Control say that only 7–8 percent of all Americans are even minimally fit. I have seen major changes just within my lifetime. When I was growing up, an hour a day of vigorous exercise was mandatory starting in the first grade and continuing all the way through high school. Today, most schools do not require or even offer any vigorous exercise at all. The only kids in high school who get any vigorous exercise are the small percentage of kids who go out for sports. The vast majority of Americans only participate in sports passively, sitting on the couch in front of the TV. Most people spend several hours every day sitting in front of a TV, playing video games, or working on a computer and sitting in front of a monitor. People drive their cars everywhere and park as close as they can to the door. And there seems to be nothing on the horizon to change the sedentary habits of Americans. Compounding the challenge, 67 percent of all Americans are overweight, and half of them are medically obese. Being overweight makes it that much harder to get off the couch and exercise, so a sedentary way of life becomes a vicious downward spiral. The less a person exercises, the fatter they get. The fatter they get, the less they feel like exercising. This is the environment in which we live: a nation of couch potatoes.

In fact, lack of fitness has become such a problem that, according to the military, 75 percent of the seventeen- to twenty-four-year-olds do not qualify for military service because they did not finish high school, have a criminal record, or *are not physically fit enough to serve.*

So much of our body and our brain is "use it or lose it." This is especially true with exercise and the Aging Challenge. First and foremost, if we do not use our muscles and our bones on a regular basis, they atrophy. Only one thing on earth builds muscles, bones, and heart muscle—lean, complete protein. But you have to give your muscles, bones, and heart muscle reason to absorb the amino acids from the lean, complete protein you eat at every meal. You need regular exercise.

Osteoporosis has reached epidemic proportions in this country. Osteoporosis is 100 percent preventable. The recipe for strong, healthy bones for life is, first and foremost, regular weight-bearing exercise like walking. Next, we need lean, complete protein at every meal. And, thirdly, there are some supplements that add that last 5 percent. But the single most important thing for strong, healthy bones is the stimulus of weight-bearing exercise. And, by the way, osteoporosis was unknown among our hunter-gatherer ancestors (Lindeberg 2010).

Cognitive decline is an accelerating problem in this country: dementia, senility, and Alzheimer's. Vigorous aerobic exercise is the single best thing you can do to keep your brain young, active, and fully functional. In fact, the only thing known to science as of this writing that stimulates neurogenesis (the creation of new brain cells) is aerobic exercise. Again, cognitive decline was unknown among our hunter-gatherer ancestors (Lindeberg 2010).

A major cause of inflammation and therefore degenerative disease is excess body fat. Regular, vigorous exercise is an integral part of the process of getting and staying lean. The lower your body fat, the lower your inflammation levels. Our hunter-gatherer ancestors were always lean and had no inflammation (Lindeberg 2010).

It is impossible to be optimally healthy without regular vigorous exercise. The most important kind of exercise is aerobic exercise, for a variety of reasons. It is the only thing that stimulates neurogenesis (the creation of new neurons or brain cells). The word "aerobic," as coined by Louis Pasteur in 1873, means "with air or with oxygen." The system that oxygenates our body is our heart, our lungs, and our circulatory system, which includes our arteries, our capillaries, and our red blood cells. Aerobic exercise puts demands on our cardiovascular system, which, over time, adapts and becomes stronger and more efficient.

A simple measure of your aerobic fitness level is your resting heart rate. As we just learned, most Americans are in lousy shape. An average American has a resting heart rate of seventy to one hundred beats per minute or even higher. A resting heart rate that high means the person has a weak heart and very little energy or endurance. What we want is a big, strong athletic heart. A *good* resting heart rate is a heart rate in the sixties. That's beats per minute. The best time to take your resting heart rate is either first thing in the morning, if you wake up naturally without an alarm clock, or just before you go to sleep.

A *very good* resting heart rate is in the fifties. And an *excellent* resting heart rate is somewhere in the forties. Not to worry. It is impossible to get your resting heart rate too low. Some world-class distance runners have resting heart rates as low as twenty-four beats per minute.

The fittest aerobic athletes in the world are cross-country skiers. They are followed by rowers. Cross-country skiing and rowing are both full-body aerobic exercises. The fundamental concept is simple: The more lean body mass you involve in your aerobic exercise, the more effective it is.

What are the benefits of full-body aerobic exercise and how does full-body aerobic exercise relate to losing weight? We have already mentioned some of the benefits of full-body aerobic exercise. Full-body aerobic exercise makes your heart bigger and stronger. That means your heart can pump out more blood per beat, so your heart does not have to beat as often or work as hard, adding years to your life and health. You can do more exercise with less effort. You are more aerobically fit. The stronger your heart, the more energy you have. Energy is a function of your heart strength. Energy is that simple and that direct. Here is simple proof. The world-record holder in the marathon runs 26.2 miles in less than two hours and four minutes. That means he is averaging 4:45 per mile for 26.2 miles. *That* is tremendous energy. His resting heart rate is twenty-four. The body does not lie.

As to other benefits, exercise is essential for muscle tone and strength. Muscles that go unused get weak and flabby. That includes our heart muscle. Aerobic exercise is essential if you want vigorous energy, stamina, and endurance. Aerobic exercise increases your HDL cholesterol, or the "good" cholesterol. HDL is the form of cholesterol that keeps the arteries of your heart clean and healthy. And the only effective way to raise your HDL cholesterol is vigorous exercise. Exercise is essential for resiliency (our ability to bounce back). Aerobic exercise is also a mood enhancer and an antidepressant. In fact, research has shown that regular aerobic exercise is often more effective in managing depression than drugs. When you do a full-body aerobic workout, your brain releases a substance called beta endogenous morphine. Beta endogenous morphine is the stuff that creates the "runner's high." In short, you will feel great after your full-body aerobic workout. And beta endogenous morphine, or endorphins for short, is one of the reasons why. Endorphins are the opposite of depression.

Aerobic exercise is also an effective stress reliever. You will find that a vigorous, aerobic workout wipes your slate clean and gives you a fresh start. Aerobic exercise is essential for a sound night's sleep. Many people who struggle with sleep find that all their sleep issues disappear when they exercise regularly and vigorously. When we do what we have evolved over millions of years to do—be physically active—we are more wide awake when we are awake and more sound asleep when we are asleep.

Specific to losing weight, full-body aerobic exercise has a whole list of benefits. First and foremost is oxygen. As we wrote in previous chapters, the technical name for fat burning is beta-oxidation. Fat requires four to five times more oxygen to be oxidized or burned than does either sugar or protein. Therefore, the more oxygen you can supply to the cells of your body, especially your muscle cells where the mitochondria burn the most fat, the more fat your body can burn. And as you get in better aerobic shape, you can burn more and more fat at higher intensities of exercise, making you a more efficient and effective fat burner.

Like most other aspects of our body, mitochondria are a use-it-or-lose-it proposition. The muscle cells of people who exercise aerobically have exponentially more mitochondria than those of sedentary people. And the more of your muscle mass you involve in your aerobic exercise, the more mitochondria you will have. Full-body aerobic exercise fully engages over 90 percent of your lean body mass. The end result? After several months of training, you will have dramatically more mitochondria, which means you will have dramatically increased your metabolism. Our body adapts to what we do on a regular basis. Remember, red blood cells carry oxygen. If you exercise aerobically on a regular basis, over time you will have more red blood cells to keep up with the demand for oxygen that exercise creates. And when you do full-body aerobic exercise, your body has to have enough red blood cells to oxygenate both your upper body and your lower body simultaneously. That takes a lot of red blood cells. After a few months of full-body aerobic exercise, you will have 20–30 percent more red blood cells. That means you can carry 20–30 percent more oxygen all the time. That means your normal daily life will become physically easy. You won't be worn out by daily life. You will breeze through your day with plenty of energy left over. You will become an active, vibrant person.

The fat burning process we discussed also includes enzymes that take part in those reactions. Again, with regular full-body aerobic exercise, there will be significantly more fat burning enzymes in your muscles cells to facilitate the fat burning (beta-oxidation) process. And remember: Mitochondria and fat burning enzymes never sleep. They are working for your benefit twenty-four hours a day. More mitochondria and more fat burning enzymes are all part of a lean, fit metabolism. It is a snowball effect. A lean, fit metabolism takes a while to get going, but once you do, it will get much easier to stay lean.

On a more basic level, part of losing weight is burning more calories than you are taking in. When you do full-body aerobic exercise, you will be amazed how many calories you will burn. If you are eating cleaner (more healthy food, less junk food) and doing full-body aerobic exercise on a regular, consistent basis, you will have shifted the energy balance equation in the direction of losing weight (body fat).

Whenever you exercise, you also speed up your metabolism. There is a unit of measure for the metabolic intensity of your exercise. It's called mets. One met is one metabolic rate. One met is your metabolism at rest: sitting in a chair or just lying in your bed. As you begin to exercise, and the intensity of your exercise increases, you are working at a higher met level. Four to five mets is a moderate aerobic exercise. Eight to ten mets is more intense. And twelve to fifteen mets is really working hard. When you elevate your metabolism like this for thirty to forty-five minutes, it takes a while for your metabolism to come back down to your resting rate again. You know you burn calories when you are exercising. If you keep your training heart rate in your optimal range, most of the calories you burn will be fat. But you may not be aware that you actually burn a significant number of calories and fat *after* your workout is over.

After you've cranked up your metabolism during your workout, it takes a while for your metabolism to settle back down to your resting state again. This is known as residual calorie burn or after-burn. The technical term for this phenomenon is called excess post-exercise oxygen consumption, or the EPOC effect. The EPOC effect is the result of the oxygen required for the processes that restore your body to a resting state and adapt your body to the exercise you just performed. Some of the changes and adaptations include hormone rebalancing, replenishment of fuel stores such as glycogen, and cellular repair. The EPOC effect includes an elevated consumption of fuel. In response to the exercise you just performed, fat stores are broken down and free fatty acids are released into your bloodstream. During recovery, more fat is burned as fuel. The EPOC effect is greatest immediately after your workout, but it lasts for a number of hours. How long the EPOC effect lasts and how much fat and how many calories you burn depend upon both the intensity and the duration of the exercise. The EPOC effect is one of the hidden bonuses of exercise. By the way, after a vigorous full-body aerobic workout, the EPOC effect can last up to twenty-four hours.

We have underscored how integral insulin management is to losing weight.

Most Americans have varying degrees of insulin resistance. Advanced insulin resistance is diabetes. As you read, seventy-nine million Americans are prediabetic. All those seventy-nine million Americans are insulin resistant. Insulin resistance means it takes progressively more insulin to clear the excess glucose from your bloodstream. In time, you wear your pancreas out, and it just cannot keep up. Then you have to go to drugs to control your insulin. Or you can exercise. By doing full-body aerobic exercise, you are making over 90 percent of your muscle mass more insulin sensitive. The more insulin sensitive your tissues are, the more easily your body handles carbohydrates and the less insulin is needed for the job. By getting in good aerobic shape, you are taking a big load off your pancreas, and you are avoiding diabetes. Between a healthy diet and full-body aerobic exercise, type 2 diabetes is both preventable and manageable drug-free. For life.

As you look at this diagram, you can see that the harder you work, the more calories you burn.

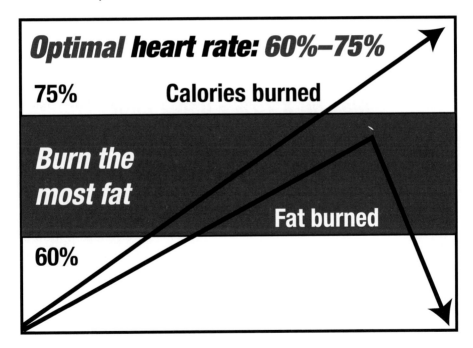

That is straightforward and intuitive. What is counterintuitive is fat burning. Notice that the fat burning arrow goes up, just like the calorie arrow. But then fat burning suddenly takes a nose dive. What's going on? The point where you see the fat burning arrow take a nose dive is the point where your body can no longer supply enough oxygen fast enough to burn fat. That point, or more accurately, that threshold, is called your anaerobic threshold. Aerobic, remember, means with air or with oxygen. Anaerobic, on the other hand, means without air. So once your training heart rate exceeds your anaerobic threshold, for all practical purposes, fat burning shuts down. The optimal training heart rate range for both aerobic fitness and for optimal fat burning is 60 to 75 percent of your maximum heart rate.

This diagram shows you how to calculate your maximum heart rate. Take 220 (which is a scientific constant) and subtract your current age. That gives you your maximum heart rate. Then multiply your maximum heart rate by 75 percent, or .75, and that gives you the upper limit of your optimal training heart rate range. Then take your maximum heart rate again and multiply it by 60 percent, or .6, and that gives you the lower limit of your optimal training heart rate range.

Training heart rate range

220 - age = maximum heart rate
Max HR X 75% = upper limit
Max HR X 60% = lower limit
*keep your training heart rate under 75%

You may be surprised how low your training heart rate range turns out to be. There is a common misconception that you have to kill yourself to get into great shape. You know the saying: No pain, no gain. That is not true. A chest-strap heart rate monitor is the single most effective tool for keeping track of your training heart rate as you work out.

Your Full-Body Aerobic Exercise Program

How do you actually do full-body aerobic exercise? As you can see in this diagram, you are going to be walking and pumping light hand-weights. The cornerstone of your exercise program is walking. This is not race walking. The optimal walking pace is 3.0 to 3.5 miles an hour. This exercise program is simple, practical, and flexible. You can walk in place at home or in your den or living room while watching TV. You can walk around your neighborhood if the weather is nice. Or you can go to a gym and walk on a treadmill. If you use a treadmill either at a gym or at home, use the manual settings. Set the speed for 3.0 miles per hour or no faster than 3.5 miles an hour. If you have access to a treadmill, take advantage of the hill feature and set the treadmill at a slight incline: three degrees to no more than five degrees. Keep the moderate speed and the slight elevation constant throughout your entire 30 to 45 minute walk.

You will be walking nonstop throughout your entire workout. You will be pumping light hand-weights. This is very important: Start with one pound (a one-pound dumbbell) in each hand. Do not start with more weight than one pound. If you are unsure of your conditioning, you may start with no weight in either hand for the first six weeks. With one pound in each hand, start walking at a comfortable pace. As you walk, pump your hand-weights. This exercise is just like normal walking, only slightly exaggerated. Take one pump per step. Every time your right hand comes up, your left foot hits the ground. Every time your left hand comes up, your right foot hits the ground. Left, right, left, right. Pump and walk, (just like in the picture of me) for two minutes.

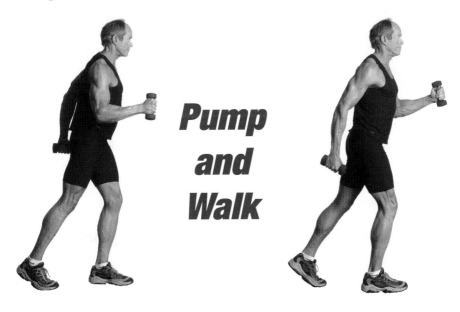

Pump and Walk

First Variation. At the end of your two-minute pump-and-walk, you are going to start doing the first of three variations. As you can see here, the first variation is called chest flyes. While walking, bring your hands up and together at chest height. Keep your elbows bent at ninety degrees and your forearms parallel to the ground. Keeping your hands at chest height, bring your elbows back as though you are trying to touch your elbows behind your back. You should feel a nice stretch in your chest muscles. If you feel strain in your shoulders, your hands are too high. Then bring your hands back together in front of you, just like in the picture. One pump per step. Every time your elbows go back, your left foot hits the ground. Every time your hands come back together in front of you, your right foot hits the ground. Left, right, left, right. Do 25 repetitions. When you have completed your 25 repetitions, go back to pumping and walking. But this time, pump and walk for only one minute.

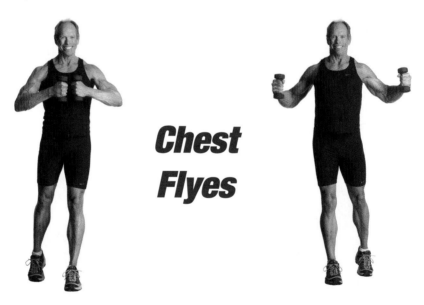

Chest Flyes

Second Variation. The second variation is known as lateral raises.

Continue to walk nonstop. Bring your hands in front of you at waist height. Your upper arms will be next to your sides and your elbows are bent at ninety degrees. Your forearms are parallel to the ground. The pivot point is at your shoulders. Lifting from your elbows, bring your arms up until your upper arms are parallel to the ground, and your forearms are parallel to each other. It is one pump per step. When your arms go up, your left foot hits the ground. When your arms come back down, your right foot hits the ground. It will look a little like you're flapping your wings. Do one set of 25 repetitions. When you have completed 25 repetitions, return to pump and walk for one minute.

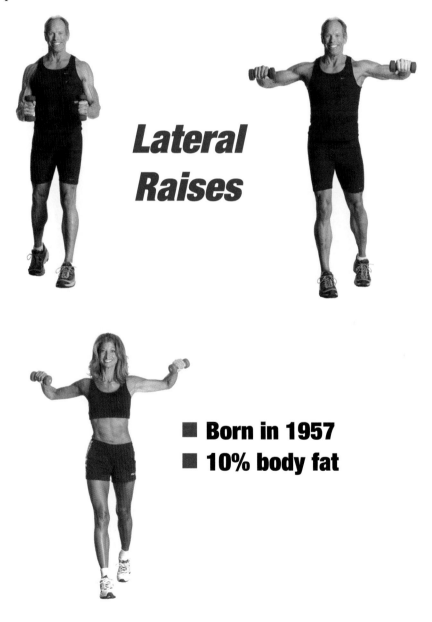

Lateral Raises

- **Born in 1957**
- **10% body fat**

Third Variation. The third variation is called overhead presses. While still walking, bring your hands up to shoulder height. Press your hands all the way up until your arms are fully extended. Then bring your hands back down to shoulder level. One pump per step. Every time your hands go up, your left foot hits the floor. Every time your hands come back down, your right foot hits the ground. Do one set of 25 repetitions. When you have completed your set of 25 repetitions, return to pumping and walking.

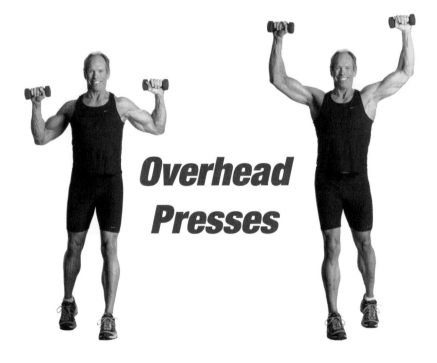

This is one full cycle, including all three variations. You will repeat the cycle over and over again throughout your entire 30 to 45 minute walk. In a 30 minute walk, you should complete four full cycles. In a 45 minute walk, you should complete six full cycles. Ideally, you should do this routine at least three days per week, but four to five is better. If you are looking for the most effective way to burn fat while you simultaneously get toned and fit, this is the exercise program for you.

How to Progress (1–5 pounds)

- ■ **Week 1 = 25 repetitions per set**
- ■ **Week 2 = 30 repetitions per set**
- ■ **Week 3 = 35 repetitions per set**
- ■ **Week 4 = 40 repetitions per set**
- ■ **Week 5 = 45 repetitions per set**
- ■ **Week 6 = 50 repetitions per set**

*Add just *one* pound every *6* weeks

As you can see on the "How to Progress" chart, on Week 1 you will do sets of 25 repetitions over and over for 30 to 45 minutes with one-pound dumbbells in each hand. The rest follows:

Week 2: Sets of 30 repetitions with one-pound dumbbells for 30-45 minutes

Week 3: Sets of 35 repetitions with one-pound dumbbells for 30-45 minutes

Week 4: Sets of 40 repetitions with one-pound dumbbells for 30-45 minutes

Week 5: Sets of 45 repetitions with one-pound dumbbells for 30-45 minutes

Week 6: Sets of 50 repetitions with one-pound dumbbells for 30-45 minutes

Once you have completed Week 6, add one more pound to each hand, so you'll have two-pound dumbbells in each hand.

Now go back to Week 1 and work your way through the six-week program again, but with two pounds in each hand. Only after you have completed each full six-week cycle do you add one more pound to each hand.

A good goal for women is to work up to three to five pounds in each hand. This will take six to nine months to achieve. Take your time. There is no rush. The important thing is to commit and follow through, doing three to five walks every week for thirty to forty-five minutes each time.

Men should also start with one pound in each hand. Work all the way through the six-week program, adding one more pound to each hand only after you have completed each full six-week program. Once you have worked all the way through the six-week program with five pounders in each hand, you may be ready to try six pounders. If you are comfortable with five pounders, that is fine. Use the weight that feels comfortable to you. If you try six pounders and you find they are comfortable, then it becomes a twelve-week process.

How to Progress (6–8 pounds)

- **Week 1-2 = 25 repetitions per set**
- **Week 3-4 = 30 repetitions per set**
- **Week 5-6 = 35 repetitions per set**
- **Week 7-8 = 40 repetitions per set**
- **Week 9-10 = 45 repetitions per set**
- **Week 11-12 = 50 repetitions per set**

Note: Add just *one* pound every *12* weeks

Men should increase the number of their repetitions every two weeks. Only add one more pound to each hand after completing the full twelve-week program. You will discover that pumping six or seven pounds non-stop for thirty to forty-five minutes is quite a workout. And it will get you into excellent condition.

Remember, walking with light hand-weights is an *aerobic* workout, *not* a weight-lifting workout. The object is *not* to see how much weight you can lift. The object is to see how smoothly and fluidly you can move while still breathing comfortably and keeping your training heart rate within your optimal range. This is the formula for success. Resist the macho trap of conventional wisdom.

What do you eat before and after your workout? It is best not to work out on an empty stomach, especially first thing in the morning. Why? You run the risk of burning off some of your precious lean body mass (muscle). What could you possibly eat at 5:30 AM or 6:00 AM in the morning, right before your workout? Half a protein shake is the perfect pre-workout meal. Mix eight to ten ounces of water or nonfat milk, one scoop of whey protein isolate, half a piece of fruit, like half a banana, blend, drink, put on your workout gear, and you are ready to roll. Whey protein is quickly and easily assimilated. Your body will suck it right up by the time you start to work out.

What should you eat post-workout to get the most out of your workout? Following exercise, there is a three-hour window technically known as your anabolic window. Right after your workout, your body is looking for things to help it rebuild and recover. During your three-hour anabolic window, your body most efficiently and effectively absorbs both protein and carbohydrates. The optimal meal immediately after your workout, even before your shower, is a full protein shake. Mix together two cups of water or nonfat milk, two scoops of whey protein isolate, and one piece of whole, fresh fruit or up to one cup of frozen, unsweetened fruit. If you want your post-workout shake thicker or colder, add ice. Blend and drink, then take your shower, get dressed, etc.

For the very best results, eat a second meal before your three-hour anabolic window closes. This meal should include a fist of lean protein, a fist of slow-burning carbs, and a thumb of healthy fat. For example, in the morning, your second meal could be an egg white omelet with spinach, mushrooms, avocado, and chicken. At lunch, your second meal could be a salad with a bed of greens like spinach, one to two medium sized boneless, skinless chicken breasts diced up over your greens, and balsamic vinaigrette dressing (only use flax seed oil or extra virgin olive oil for your oil source).

Avoid Overtraining

Exercise, especially full-body aerobic exercise, is essential to getting leaner. But more exercise is not necessarily better—and harder, more intense exercise is not necessarily better. Too much of a good thing can lead to overtraining. We overtrain any time we exceed our body's ability to recover from our last workout. If you stick with the plan I just shared, you will not overtrain. A lot of people mistakenly believe you have to do a killer workout to get into great shape. This is where a chest-strap heart rate monitor is so valuable. If you use the schedule I gave you and keep your training heart rate in the optimal range, you will get in great shape.

How do you know if you or someone else is overtraining? The first sign is excess body fat. If a person is training at the level of intensity that is appropriate for their body, they will be lean. When I see an overweight person trying to train for a marathon, I know they are asking for trouble. Or if I see an overweight person in a spin class, I know they are going to overtrain. If a person works out too hard and their training heart rate is way above their optimal range, what's going to happen? They are going to be puffing and panting. They will not burn any fat. They will just burn sugar and muscle. And when they finish their workout, they will have a ravenous appetite for carbs (sugar). So they will go home and binge on bread or cookies or crackers or pasta or cereal. Ultimately, they will just get fatter and fatter. We are not against running or weight training. But we recommend that you get lean first before you run or weight train or do anything more intense. That means men should get down to 15 percent body fat or less *before* you run or weight train. Women should get down to 22 percent body fat or less *before* you run or weight train.

Symptoms of overtraining are:

- **Increased appetite for sugar** like breads, cereals, crackers, cookies, etc.

- **Change in sleep patterns**. Either you are tired all the time and can't get enough sleep, you have trouble sleeping at all, or you are restless and suffer from insomnia.

- **You are irritable**.

- **You feel depressed**.

- **You have lost your sense of humor**.

- **Working out is not fun anymore** and you actually dread working out.

- **You get sick** with a cold or the flu.

- **You get injured**.

- **You get fatter**.

If you are measuring daily, as we recommend, you will notice that your fat is increasing and your muscle is decreasing. How can that be if you are working out? Any time you overtrain, your body will release more cortisol. Cortisol is the most powerful stress hormone your body produces. The more you overtrain, the higher your cortisol levels rise. Excess cortisol wastes away your lean body mass and facilitates fat storage. Your fat goes up and your muscle goes down. Getting fatter is one of the classic signs of overtraining.

Chapter 13

Biological Essential: Optimal Sleep

Fatigue makes cowards of us all.
—Vince Lombardi, Hall of Fame football coach

When we are trying to understand why a molecule or a behavior is essential, sometimes the most compelling argument is: What happens when you take that molecule or behavior away?

The answers are obvious with the first of our Biological Essentials: oxygen and water. Both are crucial for life—we cannot survive more than a few minutes without breathing and more than a few days without water.

The simple question to ask yourself about the Biological Essential: Optimal Sleep is: How long can you stay awake? Going one night without any sleep is not too bad. Many of us have pulled all-nighters in college or to complete a project for work. But as you well know, if you go for too many nights without sleep, you get so tired you would rather sleep than literally do anything else. In fact, sleep is so essential, and the lack of sleep so painful, that simply depriving a person of sleep is one of the most effective methods of torture used to coerce information. The person is not touched or hurt in any way. They are simply kept awake. And in a matter of just a few days, most people will say nearly anything just to get some sleep.

If sleep is so essential, how did it evolve? It is a fact that all mammals sleep. It turns out that sleep is a complex process. Sleep serves a number of functions. No one knows for sure, but there are several well-established theories on the origin and functions of sleep.

One theory that is substantiated by research is that sleep performs the functions of restoration and repair. There are two different phases of sleep: NREM (non-rapid-eye-movement) sleep and REM (rapid-eye-movement) sleep. REM sleep is when we dream. REM sleep is so essential that if you keep a person from dreaming at all, they soon become psychotic. NREM sleep serves the functions of restoration and repair of physiological functions. It is known for a fact that during NREM sleep, our body increases its rate of cell division. It is also during NREM sleep that protein synthesis takes places, including the rebuilding of our lean body mass (muscles, bones, organs, and fluids). It is also known that during NREM sleep, our immune system is strengthened and repaired.

Another theory about the evolution of sleep, known as the adaptive theory, has to do with the idea that sleep served at least two functions: the conservation of energy and protection. We adapted to sleep when it was the most hazardous to be awake (at night, when hungry predators were roaming around).

A third theory, which is also substantiated by research, is that sleep has to do with cognitive health and function. During waking hours, our brain is primarily engaged in processing a torrent of sensory information, predominantly visual stimulus. As our brain evolved into a bigger, more complex brain, we had a greater need to consolidate these sensory experiences into memories. There was the basic conflict: the processing of a nonstop torrent of incoming sensory information versus the consolidation and organization of useful experiences into long-term memories. Our brains also need to periodically refresh the circuits processing all this sensory information, just like when you hit the refresh button on your computer. By going to sleep, we shut down the flood of incoming sensory information. This gives our brains time to refresh the sensory information processing circuits and to consolidate and organize memories.

A major reason we sleep is to process information acquired during the day. And a major part of this information processing has to do with the conversion of our short-term memories into long-term memories. Eric Kandel, MD, PhD, and winner of the year 2000 Nobel Prize, has done some fundamental research on this conversion process. Dr. Kandel wrote a wonderful book, *In Search of Memory,* on our brains and memory. Dr. Kandel proved in his research that when a memory is converted from a short-term memory to a long-term memory, there is a measurable, physical, permanent change in our brain. And this conversion only happens when we sleep. As simple proof of this: When you deprive a human being of sleep, one of the first things that suffers is their memory (Kandel 2006).

Physiologically, sleep is a naturally recurring state characterized by a reduced level or absence of consciousness, the suspension of all or most sensory activity, and the inactivity of nearly all voluntary muscles. Sleep also involves lowering the body temperature. Sleep is an anabolic (building) state, which accentuates growth and rejuvenates the immune, nervous, skeletal, and muscular systems. Sleep conserves energy and actually decreases our metabolism by 5–10 percent.

There are two major types of sleep: NREM (non-rapid-eye-movement) sleep, and REM (rapid-eye-movement) sleep. NREM sleep has three stages: N1, N2, and N3. Sleep proceeds in cycles of NREM and REM. Normally the order is: N1 to N2 to N3 to N2 to REM. Each sleep cycle lasts 90 to 110 minutes. The greatest amount of N3 (the deepest sleep) occurs in the earliest cycles in our night of sleep. The amount of REM sleep increases with each succeeding sleep cycle, with the most REM sleep occurring just before natural awakening.

Stage 1 (N1) sleep refers to the transition of the brain from alpha waves (our awake state) to slower theta waves. This transition is sometimes marked by sudden twitches or jerks. We lose some muscle tone and most conscious awareness.

During Stage 2 (N2) sleep, muscular activity decreases and our conscious awareness of the external environment disappears. Stage 2 sleep occupies 45–55 percent of the total sleep of adults.

Stage 3 (N3) sleep is deep or slow wave sleep. Stage 3 sleep is characterized by delta waves, the slowest sleep waves. Stage 3 is the deepest sleep.

REM or rapid eye movement sleep accounts for 20–25 percent of the total sleep time of adults. Most memorable dreaming happens during REM sleep. In mammals, during REM sleep, there is a complete loss of muscle tone. Such paralysis may be necessary to protect us from self-damage through physically acting out scenes from the vivid dreams that occur during REM sleep.

The timing of our sleep is controlled by the circadian clock, sleep-wake homeostasis, and to a certain extent, willed behavior. As light diminishes, our brain secretes more and more melatonin (a hormone secreted by the pineal gland in our brain), until we get sleepy and go to sleep. Our circadian clock also tells us when it is time to sleep. We get into a regular rhythm of going to bed at approximately the same time and getting up at approximately the same time. It is our circadian clock that gets thrown off when we experience jet lag. Our body is telling us one thing, but our environment is telling us something else.

We evolved over millions of years to live a certain way. For millions of years, the night was dark and quiet. With the advent of agriculture, that began to change. Prior to the invention of the electric light bulb, the average American slept ten hours a night. In the twenty-first century, however, we live in a 24/7 world that never sleeps. It has never been a bigger challenge to get a sound night's sleep than now.

The criteria for an ideal environment for a sound night's sleep are: cool, dark, and quiet. A cool room is the most conducive to a sound night's sleep. The optimal temperature is 65°F. Part of the sleeping process includes lowering our body temperature. That is why we don't sleep very soundly in a hot, stuffy room. A dark room is also conducive to a sound night's sleep. Pitch black is best. Finally, a quiet room is conducive to a sound night's sleep. Make the room you sleep in as quiet as possible. Do not go to sleep with the TV on. The light from the TV will prevent the release of melatonin, and the noise and distraction will disrupt your sleep. Sometimes you may need to resort to white noise like a fan, to block out distracting environmental noise. All three factors (cool, dark, and quiet) become even more important as we age.

Optimal sleep varies according to your age. Newborns sleep up to eighteen hours out of every twenty-four. Newborns also spend almost nine hours a day in REM sleep, underscoring how essential REM sleep is to brain growth and development. A one- to three-year-old sleeps twelve to fifteen hours. Three- to five-year-olds sleep eleven to thirteen hours. For five- to twelve-year-olds, nine to eleven hours is optimal. For adolescents, nine to ten hours is optimal. For adults, including the elderly, seven to nine hours is optimal. For pregnant and lactating women, eight hours plus is optimal.

For adults, since the goal is to average somewhere between seven and nine hours out of every twenty-four hours, naps are a good way to make up for a disrupted night's sleep. Naps are an effective way to recover quickly from jet lag. This includes the so-called power nap, or a short nap of a half-hour or less, to refresh and recharge in the middle of the day; some people actually set a power nap alarm to wake themselves up after fifteen or twenty minutes so they don't go into too deep a sleep. Or a nap may involve letting yourself sleep until you wake up naturally. The length of a more natural nap will vary according to how tired you are. If you are really exhausted, you may sleep for an hour or two. If you do, it just means you really needed some sleep.

As we get older, we still need seven to nine hours of sleep; we do not need less sleep. That is a common myth. The challenge as we age is *how* to get the optimal amount of sleep, despite the difficulty sleeping we may be experiencing.

As we age, we become more glucose intolerant and more insulin resistant. One key to a sound night's sleep at any age is stable blood sugar. But increased glucose intolerance and insulin resistance means more unstable blood sugar levels. The more unstable our blood sugar, the more disrupted our sleep. When our blood sugar drops, we wake up. This is called pre-dawn syndrome. Pre-dawn syndrome is very common with alcoholics because alcoholism is sugar addiction (Larson, 1997). This is one reason drinking any kind of an alcoholic beverage with dinner or after is one the worst things you can do if you want a sound night's sleep. Alcohol may help you get to sleep, but it will cause your blood sugar to crash in the middle of the night. When your blood sugar crashes, you wake up. It is a survival mechanism.

This is also why eating a balanced meal before sleep is important if you want a sound night's sleep. The perfect pre-sleep meal includes a fist of lean protein, plus a fist of slow-burning carbohydrates, plus a thumb of raw, healthy fat, like raw nuts or raw seeds. A protein shake is a great pre-sleep meal, or consider one to two boneless, skinless chicken breasts on a bed of greens with a vinaigrette made from raw flax seed oil or olive oil and some balsamic vinegar. This will keep your blood sugar solid all night long and provide the lean, complete protein your body needs to rebuild.

Also, as you age, your body produces less melatonin. Melatonin is a hormone secreted by your brain that enables you to fall asleep and to stay asleep. Because the release of melatonin is light dependent, as light begins to dim and fade in the evening, melatonin begins to be secreted. A brightly lit environment interferes with the release of melatonin. Think back millions of years. When the sun went down, it got very dark. Our ancestors had no trouble sleeping. But sitting in a brightly lit room with the TV blasting makes it nearly impossible to release melatonin, and therefore it becomes nearly impossible to begin to feel sleepy and want to go to bed. The older you get, the more important maximizing the release of melatonin becomes. Dimming the lights as we get close to bed and doing a low-key activity like reading will help you calm down enough to feel sleepy. Taking melatonin as a supplement, especially as you get older, may also be helpful. We will talk more about melatonin and other supplements in our chapter on Supplementation.

As we age, some people feel less inclined to exercise. But consistent, vigorous exercise becomes even more important as you age. Vigorous exercise is one of the most effective behaviors to ensure a sound night's sleep.

To further underscore how essential sleep is to optimal health and losing weight, let's look at what happens when you are deprived of sleep. Here are just a few of the many symptoms of sleep deprivation:

- **Aching muscles**
- **Confusion**
- **Memory loss**
- **Headaches**
- **Increased blood pressure**
- **Increased stress hormones** (cortisol)
- **Irritability**
- **Yawning**
- **Increased risk of diabetes**
- **Excess body weight**
- **Excess body fat**
- **Obesity**

Sleep deprivation has been proven to hinder growth and the release of growth hormone. It has been proven to slow the healing process, diminish our ability to pay attention, and reduce our working memory. Sleep deprivation impairs our ability. One in every five serious motor vehicle injury accidents is caused by driver fatigue, according to the American Academy of Sleep Medicine. Eighty thousand drivers fall asleep at the wheel every day, and 250,000 traffic accidents a year are sleep-related. A study published by the *British Medical Journal* in 2000 reported that sleep deprivation has the same hazardous effects as being drunk.

When you are significantly sleep deprived, your brain automatically shuts down. You fall into a sleep state for periods ranging between a second and thirty seconds. These blackouts are called microsleeps. They are involuntary. If you nod off in front of the TV, that is one thing. But if you involuntarily nod off while driving your car, the consequences may be fatal.

Relevant to the central theme of this book, sleep deprivation can make you fatter. When you don't get an adequate amount of sound sleep, two powerful hormones are released: insulin and cortisol. Have you ever noticed that when you don't get enough sleep, you get the "munchies"? This is because lack of sleep triggers the release of insulin. The higher your insulin, the lower your blood sugar. So if lack of sleep triggers the release of insulin, your blood sugar will be driven down. Low blood sugar causes hunger. And the kinds of foods that appeal to us most when we are tired and have low blood sugar are comfort foods, especially simple and processed sugars like breads, candies, cakes, muffins, and cereals.

Another hormone that is released when you are sleep deprived is cortisol. Cortisol is the most powerful stress hormone secreted by your body. Less-than-optimal sleep is stressful (self-inflicted stress). Cortisol breaks down your lean body mass (muscle) in an effort to supply the glucose your brain has to have. Cortisol also facilitates fat storage (makes you fatter). Cortisol depresses your immune system, making you more vulnerable to colds and flu, and it compromises your ability to heal. And cortisol raises your inflammation levels.

A 2005 study (Gottlieb et al 2005) showed that people who were chronically sleep deprived were also most likely to become diabetics, in part because chronic sleep deprivation increases glucose intolerance. Glucose intolerance is a major step down the road to diabetes.

A number of studies have proven that sleep deprivation increases both food intake (you eat more when you are tired) and disrupts hormone balance (Hasler et al 2004; Gangwisch et al 2005). In fact, these studies indicate that a major cause of the obesity epidemic in the United States is chronic sleep deprivation. Sleep deprivation disrupts hormones that regulate glucose metabolism and appetite. By decreasing the hormone leptin and increasing the hormone ghrelin, sleep deprivation disrupts energy homeostasis, which leads to both increased hunger and lack of satisfaction when food is eaten.

When we don't get enough sleep, we tend to regress to self-destructive habits we are trying to avoid or overcome. When we are tired, we lose our will power. We have less resistance to temptation. This is one reason you should never shop for food when you are tired.

Bottom line: The more you sleep, the leaner you get. Optimal sleep is essential to getting leaner (burning fat and building muscle) and optimal health. It is essential if you want to feel your best, look your best, perform at your highest levels, and avoid getting sick.

When in doubt, take a nap.

Chapter 14

Biological Essential: Supplementation

I'm very excited about the idea of tuning up our biochemistry.
—Bruce Ames, PhD, Professor of Biochemistry and
Molecular Biology at the University of California, Berkeley,
international authority on aging, and author of over 500
studies on aging

Let's make our fundamental position on supplements clear right up front: Supplements are *not* substitutes. There are no substitutes for the Biological Essentials of oxygen, water, the eight essential amino acids (protein), the essential fats (especially omega-3), aerobic exercise, and sleep. That said, there are some safe and effective supplements that can enhance your health and performance, help prevent degenerative disease, and help you age more successfully.

The basic formula for an optimally healthy lifestyle is approximately 75 percent nutrition (pure water, lean protein, healthy fat, and slow-burning carbohydrates); 20 percent exercise (preferably full-body aerobic exercise), and 5 percent supplementation.

Supplementation is concerned with micronutrients as opposed to macronutrients (protein, fat, and carbohydrates). The micronutrients are the essential vitamins such as vitamin C, and essential minerals such as iron.

Among micronutrients, there is a major distinction between water-soluble vitamins and fat-soluble vitamins. Water-soluble vitamins include: vitamins B1, B2, B3, B5, B6, B12, folic acid, biotin, choline, vitamin C, inositol, PABA, and vitamin P (bioflavonoids). Fat-soluble vitamins include vitamins A, D, E, and K, and CoQ10.

Fat-soluble vitamins need the presence of fats and certain minerals to be absorbed. Fat-soluble vitamins are stored in your liver and fatty tissues. Water-soluble vitamins are not stored in your body in any significant amounts. Unused water-soluble vitamins are simply excreted in your urine. As a result, water-soluble vitamins need to be replenished every day (usually multiple times per day) to avoid depletion. And water-soluble vitamins are more easily lost in cooking.

As with any Biological Essential, one of the simplest and most graphic ways to underscore how essential a molecule is to optimal health is to see what happens when you deprive your body of that molecule. A good example is vitamin C. The molecule vitamin C is essential to human health. The disease caused by vitamin C deficiency is scurvy. Among other functions, vitamin C is essential for the formation of strong, healthy collagen. Without optimal amounts of vitamin C, the collagen your body synthesizes is too unstable to perform its function. You may not realize how important collagen is in your body until you understand the symptoms of scurvy: brown spots on the skin, spongy and bleeding gums, and bleeding from all mucous membranes. The person with scurvy looks pale, feels depressed, and is partially immobilized. As scurvy advances, there are open, suppurating wounds, loss of teeth, and eventually death. Scurvy used to be a huge problem, especially for sailors on long voyages. In 1499, the great explorer Vasco da Gama lost 116 of his crew of 170 to death from scurvy on just one voyage. In 1520, Magellan lost 208 out of the 230 men in his crew to scurvy on a single voyage.

In the mid-1700s, as an experiment, Dr. James Lind, a ship's surgeon, provided half of his ship's crew with two oranges and one lemon a day, in addition to their normal rations. The other half of the crew ate their normal rations. None of the crewmembers who received the citrus fruit got scurvy. All the other crewmembers who did not receive the citrus fruit got scurvy. In the history of science, this is considered the first controlled experiment. Dr. Lind's results proved conclusively that citrus fruit prevented scurvy. Dr. Lind published his *Treatise on the Scurvy* in 1753. As is so often the case in science, people were slow to pick up on the new paradigm. It was not until 1795 that the British Navy included lemons or limes as standard issue at sea. Limes proved to be the more popular of the two, which led to the American use of the nickname "Limeys" for British sailors.

Early in the twentieth century (1907), the concept of "vitamin" was used to describe any essential element in food that we could not do without. In 1928, a Hungarian scientist named Albert Szent-Gyorgyi, PhD, began to work intensely to identify the exact chemistry of the "vitamin" that prevented scurvy. It took Dr. Szent-Gyorgyi five years, from 1928 to 1933, to discover the substance that prevented scurvy. Late in 1933, a British chemist named Walter Norman Haworth, PhD, was able to synthesize the molecule that is now called ascorbic acid (vitamin C). By 1934, ascorbic acid (vitamin C) could be synthesized in bulk. In 1937, Dr. Haworth and Dr. Szent-Gyorgyi shared the Nobel Prize for their discovery of ascorbic acid (vitamin C). The story of vitamin C is a classic illustration of not only how long it takes for a biological problem to be solved, but also how long it takes before the new paradigm is fully accepted by the scientific community.

Another fundamental concept that is still meeting resistance is the distinction between the RDA (Recommended Daily Allowance), which is the amount of a vitamin to keep you from getting a deficiency disease, and the optimal amount of that vitamin. The objective of *optimal* amounts of a vitamin is to maximize your health, performance, life span, and health span. For example, the RDA for vitamin C is 90 mg for men and 75 mg for women. In contrast, the *optimal* intake of vitamin C is at least 3,000 mg per day.

At the root of the controversy over the difference between the RDA of a vitamin and the optimal amount of a vitamin are two different paradigms. The predominant paradigm (the Black Box of Conventional Wisdom) in this country is: If you don't have any obvious symptoms of illness, you are healthy. The predominant paradigm of health in the country is a crisis-management approach to health: Wait until you are sick, then go to heroic (and astronomically expensive) measures to merely bring you back to being symptom free. This is a mediocre response at best. The alternative paradigm is to look deeper at critical biomarkers, such as inflammation markers, to empirically measure the level of your real health, the aim being *optimal* health. Then do everything you can *now* to prevent any and all degenerative diseases, *before* you are symptomatic, and to retard the aging process as effectively as you can. One goal of this paradigm is to be drug-free and disease-free for life. This alternative paradigm is a preventive or proactive approach to life and health, meaning you should do everything you can *now* to prevent crises in the future. And if you do a good enough job, you may be able to avoid any major health crises and die of old age in your nineties or older.

To give you some perspective on the difference between the RDA and optimal amounts of a vitamin, let's look at vitamin C as an example. Most animals are able to synthesize vitamin C in their bodies. Our ancient ancestors lost the ability to synthesize vitamin C somewhere between fifty-eight and sixty-five million years ago. One theory is that the fruits and vegetables then were so rich in vitamin C that it was (from an evolutionary point of view) a waste of resources to synthesize something so readily available. Unfortunately, in our modern obesogenic environment, that has drastically changed. One strong argument is that we actually thrive on a much higher intake of vitamin C, rather than the amounts prescribed by the RDA. These *optimal* levels are based on the estimates of the intake of vitamin C among hunter-gatherer societies, who ate real, natural foods. Hunter-gatherers routinely took in several thousand milligrams of vitamin C per day versus the 90 mg recommended for men by the RDA. And, as you have learned, hunter-gatherers suffered from virtually no degenerative disease (Lindeberg 2010).

Another argument favoring higher intakes of vitamin C is the amount of vitamin C that animals routinely produce. Goats, for example, typically produce 13,000 mg of vitamin C (ascorbic acid) every single day. And when goats are under stress, they produce as much as 29,000 mg of vitamin C per day.

What is also interesting to note, from an evolutionary point of view, is that bone analysis reveals no vitamin or mineral deficiencies in our hunter-gatherer ancestors. Bear in mind, the ancestral hunter-gatherer diet was predominantly wild game meat that was lean, fresh, and rich in nutrients, including omega-3 essential fat. The only carbohydrates our ancestors ate were fresh fruits and vegetables. And the only thing our ancestors drank was water. Our ancestors only ate highly nutritious foods. Our ancestors never ate any toxic or processed foods that robbed their bodies of essential nutrients the way the majority of today's processed foods do. And the foods our ancestors ate were far more nutritious than our foods today because the soil in which our ancestors' foods grew was never depleted, and our ancestors' food was never mass-produced. The foods our ancestors ate were fresh every single day. As a result, our hunter-gatherer ancestors were lean, vigorously healthy, and had no deficiencies or degenerative diseases. Of course, all that began to slowly change with the advent of the agricultural revolution.

When it comes to development, growth requires even more high-quality nutrition. This is why pregnant and lactating women need an even more nutritious diet than the rest of us. And we know what happens to a fetus if the mother was undernourished or malnourished—underweight babies, locked into survival mode, destined for significant degenerative disease as they grow into middle and old age. Because they are growing, children also require extra nutrition: 50 percent more lean, complete protein and 50 percent more essential (omega-3) fat, plus a broad spectrum of vitamins and minerals. The time spent in the womb and early childhood are irreplaceable windows of opportunity to optimize nutrition and growth. Once that window closes, it is closed forever.

Unfortunately, we live in an obesogenic environment. So much of the food available today is empty, meaning it has no nutritional value at all. In fact, many processed foods today are so nutritionally incomplete that they literally rob our bodies of nutrition. Biochemical reactions in our body require specific components in order to take place. If any one of these components is not present in the food itself, our body will rob itself to complete these reactions to metabolize that empty food. The result is that the majority of Americans suffer from varying degrees of malnutrition. As an example, many metabolic processes require B-complex vitamins. Processed foods, made out of white sugar and white flour, contain no or virtually no B-complex vitamins. And don't be fooled by the word "enriched." "Enriched" is a Black Box of Conventional Wisdom word. Scientifically, "enriched" means that the food manufacturer takes *all* of the vitamins and minerals out of the food (such as in the case of white flour), and then adds back in a *trace* of the former vitamin and mineral content that was originally in that food, then calls this empty food "enriched."

Unfortunately, most people perceive "enriched" as giving them more vitamins and minerals than were there originally. Enriched is yet another entry in the long list of word games food manufacturers play to deceive us into thinking we are eating something healthy, when in fact, we are eating empty food that has had virtually all the nutrition processed out of it. As a result, when people eat these empty calories, they are literally a net loss.

Then, to compound this problem, because of the requirement for extended shelf life, all the raw, healthy fats have been replaced with hydrogenated fats and trans fats. Hydrogenated and trans fats are worse than nutritionally empty; they fill the receptor sites on our cell membranes reserved for essential omega-3 fat, which then interferes with our fundamental biology and is therefore literally toxic to our body. Our modern obesogenic diet with its massive sugar content and toxic fats is a far cry from the completely natural, highly nutritious diet of our ancestors.

As we age, getting optimal nutrition becomes an even bigger challenge. As we age, we have a harder time absorbing and assimilating nutrients. As a result, the vitamin and mineral intake for older people should actually be increased. And yet, the diets of a lot of older people are sorely lacking.

There have now been decades of research on the aging process. One of the pioneers in the area of aging and nutrition is Dr. Denham Harman. Dr. Harman has been researching aging for a very long time. Dr. Harman received his PhD in chemistry from the University of California, Berkeley. Then he realized that in order to truly understand aging, he needed to learn more biology. So, after working in the world of chemistry for a number of years, Dr. Harman received his MD from Stanford University Medical School. In between his internship and his residency in internal medicine, he worked in a research lab at U.C. Berkeley. There, he was able to intensely pursue the puzzle of aging. After months of research, he came upon the idea of free radical damage as the cause of aging. With the use of antioxidants, he was able to increase the average life expectancy of mice by 30 percent.

In 1958, Dr. Harman became the chairman of the department of cardiovascular research at the University of Nebraska, College of Medicine. In 1961, Dr. Harman published a study that proved that processed fats dramatically increased the cancer rate in mice. In 1968, Dr. Harman published a study using even more advanced antioxidants that increased the average life span of mice by 45 percent. But he was still frustrated because he felt he had not yet solved the aging puzzle. Then he discovered that many of the free radicals in your body are produced by your mitochondria. In 1972, he published a paper called *The Mitochondrial Theory of Aging*. Born in 1916,

Dr. Harman, MD, PhD, is still doing research. At ninety-five years of age, he is still five feet, ten inches tall, weighs the same 140 pounds he always has, and remains an avid walker.

Bruce Ames, PhD, full professor of biochemistry and molecular biology at the University of California, Berkeley, is another major proponent of the free radical theory of aging and mitochondrial damage. Dr. Ames has been studying aging for over sixty years. Dr. Ames got on the trail that Dr. Harman had blazed and took it even further. Dr. Ames studied the mitochondria of rats. He noticed that the mitochondria of old rats consumed less oxygen, had stiffer membranes, and shuffled electrons less efficiently. He also noticed that the mitochondria of old rats made a lot more oxidants (free radicals). Because Dr. Ames' wife (who is also a biochemist) is Italian, they have a second home in Italy. In the 1990s, acetyl-L-carnitine was being sold as a "pick me up" in Italy, and this piqued the Ames' curiosity.

Dr. Ames decided to test acetyl-L-carnitine, a nutrient that transports fatty acids across lipid membranes into the mitochondria to be burned as fuel. Dr. Ames reasoned that high levels of acetyl-L-carnitine might combat the problem of aging membranes and decrepit enzymes. Within weeks, the improvement in the animals' biochemistry and behavior was dramatic. Their mitochondria were going full bore, and they had become far more active. But the old rats were still churning out free radicals—in fact, at an even faster rate. This was the first step in his research.

Dr. Ames then decided to add an agent to neutralize the oxidants. He tried R-lipoic acid, which is a mitochondrial antioxidant. The results were profound. The oxidants and the oxidative damage to mitochondrial components dropped dramatically. Both the structure and the function of the mitochondria improved. This demonstrated that the combination of the nutrient (acetyl-L-carnitine) and the antioxidant (R-lipoic acid) have a synergistic effect. The two together are better than either one alone. And as a bonus, there were exciting changes in the old rats' brains. Their memories improved so much that they were almost as fast as the young rats. Dr. Ames is hopeful that his team's studies of the effects of dietary supplements in aging rats could lead to a new appreciation of the power of nutrition (versus drugs). He's very excited about the idea of tuning up our biochemistry. Born in 1928, Dr. Ames says he has no interest in retiring; he is still trim and fit and having too much fun with his research.

Dr. Ames' most recent research (2006) was revealed in his paper on the *Triage Theory of Aging*. Triage is the process of sorting tasks or actions according to a system of priorities. Triage is often applied in emergency medical situations, where the most seriously wounded are treated first. According to Dr. Ames' theory, Nature (evolution) prioritizes available resources. If some resources are scarce, evolution will always choose short-term gains over the long-term investment. For example, when the fetus in the womb is faced with limited resources, it opts for a smaller body size and a quicker delivery in an effort to survive and potentially reproduce. Evolution always opts for short-term survival with the chance of reproduction over a long-term investment in maintenance and repair.

In the case of micronutrients, your body will take limited resources and use them to nourish your brain and heart first, so you can survive. What gets short-changed is the protection and repair of your DNA. For example, if there is a shortage of iron in your body, your heart gets it first, because if your heart does not get adequate iron, you die. Early and lifelong deficiencies of micronutrients, such as iron, copper, or B-complex vitamins, show up as degenerative disease down the road, including diseases like cancer and Alzheimer's. Lack of optimal micronutrient resources accelerates the aging process.

The key interface in our body is the cell membrane, both of cells themselves and the membranes of the organelles, such as mitochondria. The health and permeability of the cell/organelle membrane determines how easily and efficiently nutritious elements get in and toxins are expelled.

Because of the crucial importance of the cell membranes, the most important supplement you can take is omega-3 essential fat (molecularly distilled fish oil capsules). This will help balance your ratio of omega-3 to omega-6 fatty acids, which as you learned previously, is often heavily tilted toward omega-6 fatty acids. Omega-3 is difficult to get in our culture. Salmon only provides a meager supply of omega-3, even if you ate salmon every day. Raw flax seeds and raw flax seed oil are substantial sources of omega-3, but they are challenging to get and impractical to use in our busy lives. Molecularly distilled fish oil capsules offer the highest quality source of omega-3 in a practical format. Simply take six to twelve capsules a day. I personally take six capsules of omega-3 in the morning with my breakfast shake and six more capsules in the evening with my pre-sleep meal. We will teach you how to determine how much you need in our chapter "Listen to YOUR Body."

Why is taking molecularly distilled fish oil capsules so important? Omega-3 is important because omega-3 fat is the primary component of every membrane of every single cell in your body. This includes the membranes of the hundreds of mitochondria in each and every one of your cells. Neither your mitochondria nor your trillions of cells can thrive without a generous amount of omega-3 fat.

You will also recall from the chapter on the Inflammation Challenge that molecularly distilled fish oil capsules are the single most powerful anti-inflammatory you can take. We think you will find molecularly distilled fish oil capsules a safe and effective supplement for you and your family. The benefits, short-term and long-term, are huge.

In addition, one of the factors that drives hunger is called deficiency hunger. Your body needs certain essential molecules. When you consistently supply your body with the Biological Essentials it needs, you feel satisfied. But if you eat a lot of processed fats or trans fats, for example, neither of these supplies any essential fat. In fact, processed fats and trans fats fill essential fat receptor sites, leaving your body hungry for what it really needs. Your body will continue to hunger for the missing essentials and drive you to eat more and more food in an effort to acquire those essentials. This is called deficiency hunger. Deficiency hunger applies to all the Biological Essentials, including essential fat (omega-3), vitamins, and minerals.

The next most important supplement after omega-3 is a high-potency, high-quality, broad-based multivitamin and multi-mineral. You want a multi that offers significantly more of every nutrient than the RDA. Again, our goal is *optimal* health and performance, not mere survival. Also, bear in mind Dr. Ames' research on triage. For optimal health and for maximum life and health span, we need to provide optimal micronutrient nutrition our entire lives. A high-potency, high-quality multi should include all the vitamins, especially all the B-complex vitamins, as well as all the essential minerals, including all the trace minerals. It is impossible to combine all these micronutrients in one small pill. A high-quality multi will require you to take multiple tablets. The multi that Sandy and I take every day requires nine tablets (three tablets, three times per day)—just for our multi. A high-quality multi tablet should dissolve very quickly in a glass of vinegar. Cheap multi-vitamins often come in hard shells that our bodies have a tough time breaking down. A high-quality multi is simply high-potency vitamin/mineral powders pressed together that readily dissolve in your stomach.

Once we cover all the basics with our high-quality, high-potency multivitamin/multi-mineral and omega-3 supplements, we turn to the antioxidants. Recall that free radical damage is a fundamental component of the aging process and of degenerative disease. Antioxidants are molecules that donate electrons to neutralize free radicals. The development of antioxidants was part of the initial adaptation to a more oxygen-rich environment, billions of years ago. But if your internal antioxidant system is overwhelmed due to your poor diet, lack of sleep, lack of exercise, use of alcohol, the aging process, and stress, then your body is in oxidative stress. Oxidative stress accelerates the aging process and lays the groundwork for degenerative disease. The answer? Be proactive.

Vitamin C is the most effective water-soluble antioxidant. For best results, take vitamin C multiple times a day. Vitamin C is crucial to the health of your collagen. Collagen is integral to so many components of your body that if you don't get enough vitamin C, your collagen fails and you die. Vitamin C is also foundational to your immune system. If you want to avoid colds and flu and be optimally healthy, you need plenty of vitamin C. Vitamin C is also a powerful anti-inflammatory.

How much vitamin C? A good goal is 3,000 milligrams per day (in addition to the vitamin C in your multi). Again, vitamin C is water-soluble. Any vitamin C you don't use just gets excreted. Vitamin C is very safe. Secondly, because vitamin C is water-soluble, spread it out throughout your day for best results. As Dr. Linus Pauling, PhD, biochemist and the only winner of two unshared Nobel Prizes, said, "What matters is the average level of vitamin C in your blood over a twenty-four-hour period." I personally take significantly more than 3,000 mg of vitamin C per day, but 3,000 mg is a good goal.

Ideally, we want to protect all of our tissues from the ravages of free radicals. In order to provide complete protection, we need to take both water-soluble and fat-soluble antioxidants. Perhaps the most effective fat-soluble antioxidant is vitamin E. Protecting the membranes of our cells and our organelles (especially the membranes of our mitochondria) is crucial to attaining and sustaining optimal health. Since all membranes are made out of phospholipids (essential fats), the only kind of antioxidant that can protect our cell membranes from free radical damage is a fat-soluble antioxidant. Vitamin E is also important to heart health. Being a fat-soluble antioxidant, simply take one 400 IU (international unit) pill of *gamma* tocopherol in the morning with your breakfast shake. This is an enhanced mix of tocopherols.

What about supplementation to enhance weight loss? First and foremost, you need to satisfy your body's essential biological needs in order to eliminate deficiency hunger. This starts with six to twelve capsules of molecularly distilled fish oil. Next, your supplement routine needs to include a high-potency multivitamin/multi-mineral and some additional antioxidants (vitamin C and gamma E).

Then, since the key is the health and efficiency of your mitochondria, the more mitochondria you have, the faster and more efficient your metabolism. The only effective way to increase the number of mitochondria is exercise. The more lean body mass you include in your aerobic exercise, the more mitochondria you will have. Full-body aerobic exercise stimulates mitochondria growth in over 90 percent of your lean body mass. The next factor is the health and vitality of each mitochondrion.

As we learned from Dr. Bruce Ames, PhD, the two most effective supplements for stimulating and rejuvenating mitochondria are acetyl-L-carnitine and R-lipoic acid. Remember, acetyl-L-carnitine facilitates the transport of free fatty acids (fat) into your mitochondria to be burned as fuel. R-lipoic acid (the "R" form is the biologically active form of lipoic acid) acts as a mitochondrial antioxidant; the synergy of these two supplements (taking them together) dramatically enhances the actions of your mitochondria. This includes the mitochondria of your brain, which results in a brighter, more active memory. R-lipoic acid is processed through your body fairly quickly. So for best results, take one 300 mg capsule of R-lipoic acid along with one 500 mg capsule of acetyl-L-carnitine several times a day. This will not only enhance your body's ability to burn fat, it will enhance your brain and significantly slow the aging process.

What about bone health at any age, but particularly as we get older? Most of us understand the importance of calcium to bone strength and health. But strong, healthy bones are more complicated than simply taking some calcium. The single most important factor in strong, healthy bones is weight-bearing exercise. Walking is a weight-bearing exercise. Swimming is not a weight-bearing exercise. Walking and pumping light hand-weights will stimulate your entire skeleton.

Next, you need the eight essential amino acids (protein) to build the collagen that provides the scaffolding in your bones upon which your body hangs calcium. You can't store protein. That is one reason you need to eat a fist of lean, complete protein with every one of your four to six meals a day.

The next factor for strong, healthy bones is vitamin D3. Vitamin D3 is a fat-soluble vitamin that is actually a hormone. Vitamin D3 has a number of functions, one of which is to enable your body to absorb calcium and use that calcium to effectively build and maintain bones. According to a recent study (Ginde et al 2009) nearly 50 percent of all Americans have suboptimal levels of Vitamin D3. Vitamin D3 is fat-soluble, so you only need to take one small capsule each morning with your breakfast shake. We recommend one 5,000 IU capsule of vitamin D3.

Next, you need a form of calcium your body can actually assimilate. Calcium citrate is the easiest for your body to assimilate. But to get the most out of your calcium, you need to take magnesium citrate. Calcium and magnesium work together in a 2:1 ratio: two parts calcium citrate to one part magnesium citrate.

How much calcium citrate and how much magnesium citrate should you take? We suggest 1,200 mg of calcium citrate combined with 600 mg of magnesium citrate. Calcium citrate usually comes in 200 mg capsules so that means six capsules per day. Magnesium citrate usually comes in 160 mg capsules, so that means four capsules per day. An easier way to take your calcium/magnesium is to take half of the combination in the morning with your breakfast shake and the other half in the evening with your pre-sleep meal.

CoQ10 is another fat-soluble antioxidant. CoQ10 is optional, but the reason we mention it is because CoQ10 is found primarily in the inner membranes of your mitochondria. CoQ10 is a component of the electron transport chain and participates in aerobic cellular respiration, generating energy in the form of ATP. Ninety-five percent of all the energy in your body is generated this way. As a result, the organs with the highest energy requirements in your body, such as your heart, liver, and kidneys, have the highest concentrations of CoQ10· CoQ10 also has the ability to give and receive electrons, and because of this unique ability, CoQ10 protects the lipids in the mitochondrial membrane from being oxidized. CoQ10 also prevents the oxidation of bases, particularly in mitochondrial DNA. CoQ10 also has the ability to regenerate other antioxidants such as vitamin E, so your body can use them over and over again. And circulating CoQ10 prevents LDL cholesterol (the "bad" cholesterol) from being oxidized and so helps prevent cardiovascular disease. Because CoQ10 is fat-soluble, we recommend one 200 mg capsule with your breakfast shake in the morning.

As we get older, our joints sometimes bother us. The combination of glucosamine and chondroitin can be helpful for joint health. Together, these nutrients have been found to help regenerate cartilage. Take one capsule (each capsule contains 400 mg of glucosamine sulfate and 450 mg of chondroitin sulfate) in the morning with your breakfast shake and one capsule at night with your pre-sleep meal. This combination is even more effective if you take it with a powerful anti-inflammatory such as omega-3 fish oil capsules.

There is a common misconception that as we get older, we need less sleep. That is not true. Even as we age, we still need seven-plus hours of sleep per night on the average. However, as some people age, they have a harder time getting to sleep and/or staying asleep. One of the reasons may be melatonin. Melatonin is a natural hormone that is secreted by the pineal gland in your brain. When we are young, most of us produce plenty of melatonin. But, as is often the case, as we get older, some of us produce less than we need. Melatonin has been found to help most people get to sleep more easily and stay asleep longer. Melatonin is also useful to help reset your internal clock (circadian rhythm) when it has been thrown off by jet lag.

In addition to being an effective supplement to help anyone of any age get to sleep and stay asleep, melatonin is also one of the most powerful antioxidants. Melatonin has the ability to cross membranes, including the blood/brain barrier. As a result, melatonin's primary role seems to be the protection of both our nuclear and our mitochondrial DNA from oxidative stress. As such, melatonin has important anti-aging properties. Melatonin protects your brain, enhances your memory, and acts as a powerful anti-inflammatory.

Melatonin also has weight-loss benefits. Melatonin is involved in energy metabolism and weight control. Melatonin promotes the recruitment of brown adipose tissue and enhances its activity. Brown adipose tissue, or so-called brown fat, is much more metabolically active than regular body fat. Eskimos have a lot of brown fat to keep them warm. The effect of melatonin on brown fat raises your basal metabolic rate by stimulating thermogenesis (heat generation) in the mitochondria. Thus, you burn more fat and more calories twenty-four hours a day.

The most effective way to use melatonin is to start with one 3 mg capsule of sustained-release melatonin. Take the single capsule at the start of your pre-sleep meal thirty to sixty minutes before you intend to turn out the light to go to sleep. Eat your meal. Brush and floss. Get in bed and read until you feel drowsy. With the first wave of drowsiness, set down your book, turn off your light, get into your favorite sleeping position, and relax into a sound night's sleep.

How do you know if one 3 mg capsule is optimal for you? When you first begin to take melatonin, you may experience a couple of things. Sometimes people dream a lot the first few nights. This is not unusual. It just means your brain is catching up on REM sleep. Sometimes people sleep longer than they expected. This just indicates that you were more tired than you thought you were. Some people feel a little groggy the first morning or two. Again, this may just be your brain catching up on sleep. If by the third or fourth morning, you still feel groggy, then maybe one 3 mg capsule is a little too much melatonin. Cut back to 1 mg or 2 mg. Within a week or so of trial and error, you will find the amount of melatonin that is optimal for you.

On the other hand, some people don't experience any initial benefit. This may mean that one 3 mg capsule is not enough melatonin. Simply increase from one 3 mg capsule to two 3 mg capsules for a total of 6 mg. Again, you should find the optimal amount for your brain dialed in within a week or so. By the way, 6 mg is still a very safe and conservative amount of melatonin. In research studies, doctors have given cancer patients 50 mg a night with great results. Again, you will have the best results with sustained-release melatonin.

As we said, supplements are not meant to be substitutes for the basics of water, protein, healthy fat, slow-burning carbs, exercise, and sleep. But as Dr. Ames said, low-grade malnutrition can accelerate the aging process and leave you vulnerable to degenerative disease. Start with the essentials: omega-3 fish oil capsules; a high-quality, broad-based multivitamin/multi-mineral; and vitamins C and E. The other supplements can be taken if and when they make sense to you. It is best to take supplements with food and plenty of water.

Recommended Supplements:

- **Omega-3 (molecularly distilled fish oil)**: 1,000 mg per capsule (350 mg of EPA and 250 mg of DHA), 6-12 Caps, spread out in 2-3 doses

- **High-quality multi-mineral/multivitamin**: 3 tabs, 3 times per day

- **Vitamin C**: 1,000 mg, 3 times per day

- **Gamma E**: 400 IU, 1 time per day

- **Acetyl L-Carnitine**: 500 mg/**R-Lipoic Acid** 300 mg, taken together, twice per day

- **Calcium Citrate/Magnesium Citrate**: 2:1 ratio (1,200 mg of calcium to 600 mg of magnesium), spread out in two to three doses

- **Vitamin D3**: 5,000 IU, once per day

- **Melatonin** (sustained-release): As needed for sleep

Optional:

- **Glucosamine/Chondroitin sulfate**: (400 mg/450 mg respectively), one capsule, twice per day

- **CoQ10**: 200 mg, once per day

Refer to the Resources to find where you can order these. Additional recommended supplements will also be listed, should you decide you would like to further enhance your health and/or address specific issues.

Section Three

Effective Actions

Chapter 15

Set YOUR Personal Goals

If you don't know where you're going, any road will get you there.
—Lewis Carroll (1832-1898),
Alice's Adventures in Wonderland, 1865

In Sections One and Two, we discussed your challenges and the essential components of optimal health and effective weight (fat) loss. This next section will spell out precisely *what to do* to effectively lose weight (fat) and *how to do it.* We begin with a conceptual framework for our Effective Actions. As you read, keep this list of basic concepts in mind:

Fundamental Concepts:

- **Optimal Hydration**
- **Consistently Stable Blood Sugar**
- **Full Body Aerobic Exercise**
- **Optimal Sleep**
- **Listen to YOUR Body**

The above concepts are prioritized based upon several criteria: first and foremost, the health and needs of your brain; secondly, the requirements of optimal health; and thirdly, the requirements of effective weight (fat) loss.

If we next translate the five fundamental concepts into five effective actions, we get the following prioritized list:

Effective Actions

- **For optimal hydration**, drink at least 8–12, eight-ounce glasses of pure water every day. One gallon is even better.

- **At each of your four to six daily meals**, have a shake or eat a fist of lean, complete protein; plus a fist of slow-burning, low glycemic load carbohydrates; plus a thumb of healthy fat.

- **For exercise**, walk with light hand-weights for 30–45 minutes, 3 to 5 times per week.

- **For optimal sleep**, average 7–9 hours of sleep every night.

- **To listen to YOUR body**, measure your weight, your waist, your navel skinfold, and your thigh skinfold every morning and write it down.

Effective Actions

1. Drink more pure *water*

2. Eat 4-6 Meals: Ideally a breakfast shake + 1-2 caps, post-workout shake + 1-2 caps, plus 3-4 meals of a fist + fist + 1-2 caps

3. *Walk* with light hand-weights for 30-45 minutes, 3 to 5 times a week

4. *Sleep* 7 to 9 hours a night

5. *Measure:* weigh, measure waist, measure navel and thigh skinfold

---

These five actions form the core of a lifestyle that will enable you to overcome the challenges you face so you can consistently meet and exceed your body's molecular imperatives. As a result, you will be able to effectively lose body fat, enhance your lean body mass, and get leaner. And the leaner you get, the better you will look, the better you will feel, the more energy you will have, and the more attractive you will be.

Set YOUR Personal Goals

As with any journey, you need to have a clearly defined destination, an accurate road map, and a well-thought-out itinerary to get you to your destination on time.

The process by which we define our destination is called goal setting. Each of us only has a finite amount of time and energy. One of the biggest challenges in life is deciding how you are going to spend your time and your energy. No one can do it all. No one can have it all. We have to make choices. Setting a goal is a way of making those choices. A goal is a target. A goal is a way to focus your energy so you are more effective at getting what you want. Along with a clearly defined, positive, measurable goal, you need a deadline, and you need a step-by-step action plan that will get you to your goal. In this chapter, we will explain how to set your outcome goal, your process goals, and your performance goals.

Your number one goal is to achieve your ideal body weight. As you learned in the chapter on the Body Composition Challenge, the only accurate way to determine your true ideal body weight is to do a seven-site skinfold body composition test. This first test establishes your baseline. You will subsequently test your body composition to analyze your progress and fine-tune your process. You will need a skinfold caliper and someone to help you measure a couple of hard-to-reach sites. Please refer to our website (www.TheJoeDillonDifference.com) to see exactly how and where to take your seven-site skinfold measurements. Enter in all your data on our website and print out your result. On the bottom of your results, you will see your true ideal body weight. If you recall, your true ideal body weight is your lean body mass (your muscles, bones, organs and the fluids of your body—your fat-free weight) plus an optimal amount of body fat (15 percent or less for men and 22 percent or less for women). In the chapter, "Listen to YOUR Body," we will share with you how to calculate your ideal weight if you already have less than 15 percent or 22 percent body fat.

You will have your own unique outcome goals. Perhaps you want to get leaner. Perhaps you want to improve in an athletic event. Perhaps you want to increase muscle. What matters is that you not only have a goal, but also a realistic time frame in which you can attain that goal. Let's consider an average American woman. The average American woman weighs 138 pounds and has 36 percent body fat and is five feet, five inches tall. Her ideal body weight would be 113.38 pounds based on her lean body mass of 88.44 pounds plus an optimal body fat of 22 percent.

To reach 22 percent body fat and her ideal weight of 113 pounds, she would have to lose approximately 25 pounds of fat. Given that a woman can only lose somewhere between a half-pound and one pound of fat per week, that means it will take our average American woman somewhere between twenty-five to fifty weeks to reach her ideal body weight.

That's a long time, so it makes sense to break her ultimate outcome goal of 113 pounds and 22 percent down to three-month or twelve-week intermediate goals. First, by breaking down a bigger, more ambitious goal into smaller, bite-sized chunks, it makes the whole goal more approachable. Keep in mind that, although you will want to weigh yourself daily, we are talking about *fat loss* here, not indiscriminate *weight loss*. Ideally, our average American woman will gain some muscle as she gets leaner. This will change her ultimate goal weight upward, but that will not change her need to lose 25 pounds of fat. *A loss on the scale is meaningless unless your other measurements are coming down as well.* This is why it will be important to monitor your body fat percentage on a regular basis, so you will always know you are losing fat and not lean mass. In "Listen to YOUR Body," we will explain this in more detail.

A realistic twelve-week initial outcome goal would be to weigh 132 pounds and lose six pounds of fat (to be conservative), or half a pound of fat per week. If she gained two pounds of muscle, she will have only lost four pounds *on the scale*, but she would still be right on track. It is essential that she do her seven-site skinfold body composition test every week. As we described above, she will adjust her daily process (lean protein, slow-burning carbs, essential fat, exercise, sleep, etc.), so she stays on course to lose fat and gain muscle. This is why weekly seven-site body composition tests are so important. If you don't test every week and measure every morning, you are traveling without plotting your course on your map. You are flying blind.

At the end of the first twelve weeks, it is time to reevaluate and set her next intermediate outcome goal. She would compare her initial body composition test (her baseline) to her results at twelve weeks. What has happened to her body fat percentage? Has it gone down? What has happened to her fat weight? Has it gone down? And what has happened to her lean body mass? Has it increased slightly? Based on her actual results at the twelve-week mark, she will adjust her outcome goal. For example, if she has gained some muscle, this will raise her ideal body weight at 22 percent. Her seven-site body composition test will spell out exactly what her new ideal weight at 22 percent body fat will be.

She will continue this twelve-week process, constantly testing and adjusting her daily process based on her daily measurements and her weekly seven-site skinfold body composition test. If she sticks with The Joe Dillon Difference lifestyle and constantly measures and tests, she will never get lost or distracted. She will hone in on her ideal body weight and achieve it on or before schedule.

An outcome goal defines your ultimate destination. It is wise to create *initial, intermediate,* and *ultimate* outcome goals when you are goal setting. How you achieve these goals is through the use of *process goals*. And how you measure your progress is through the use of *performance goals*. Therefore, if you change your outcome goals, both your process and your performance goals will change accordingly.

The following are some examples of process goals for our average American woman. The idea is to create an enjoyable, sustainable process that makes your ultimate outcome goal inevitable. If you put together an effective process, you will not only reach your outcome goal of your ideal weight, you will be able to maintain your ideal weight for the rest of your long and much healthier life.

- **Drink at least an ounce of pure water for every two pounds of body weight**: 138 divided by 2 equals 69 ounces, or 8.63 eight-ounce glasses per day. So a good process goal would be to drink 8 to 12, eight-ounce glasses of pure water every day.

- **Eat at least 1 to 1.5 grams of lean protein per pound of body weight.** To protect her lean body mass and give her body the raw material to build more muscle, bone, and heart muscle, she needs to consistently intake an optimal amount of pure protein. At 138 pounds and 36 percent body fat, she needs at least 138 grams of pure protein per day. Given her body fat percentage, she is probably glucose intolerant and insulin resistant, so she will need an

additional 50 percent more pure protein to keep her blood sugar
stable and avoid insulin spikes, thus 138 pounds times 1.5 equals
207 grams of pure protein. If we divide 207 grams of pure protein by five or six small meals per day, it means she needs to eat
somewhere between thirty-five and forty grams of pure protein per
meal to achieve her optimal protein intake. As examples of what
this looks like, one medium boneless, skinless chicken breast (or
about 3.5 to 4 ounces cooked) will yield approximately twenty-
five grams of pure protein. To reach thirty-five to forty grams of
pure protein, she will have to eat about 1.5 medium-sized chicken
breasts per meal, or about five to six ounces. As an alternative, she
could drink a protein shake as a meal and include about 1.5 to 2
scoops of whey protein isolate.

■ **Keep her carb intake down to 100 grams of carbohydrates
per day.** Make them low glycemic load carbohydrates, like no
more than one to two cups of vegetables per meal or one medium-sized apple per meal.

■ **For essential fat, take six to twelve capsules of molecularly distilled fish oil per day.** To slow the assimilation of carbohydrates and keep her blood sugar stable, with each meal, eat a
thumb of healthy fat (e.g., ten to twelve raw almonds, or one slice
of avocado, etc.).

■ **Schedule in her full-body aerobic exercise program.** To stimulate her metabolism and to enhance her lean body mass (muscle),
her process goal for exercise might be to walk with light hand-
weights for 30 to 45 minutes, three to five times each week.

■ **Get ample sleep per night.** Her process goal for sleep might be
to get at least seven hours of sound sleep each night.

■ **Take her supplements each day.** Her process goal for supplements might be to take her supplements every morning with her
breakfast shake, including her omega-3 capsules, and her additional supplements with her other meals.

■ **Take her four basic measurements each morning: weight,
waist, navel, and thigh skinfold.**

One helpful way of organizing process goals is to create a daily log. The following are examples of things she wants to keep track of on a daily basis to ensure she achieves her ultimate goal.

- **Number of eight-ounce glasses of water per day** (process goal: a minimum of 8–12, eight-ounce glasses per day).

- **Total grams of pure protein per day** (process goal: 207 grams of pure protein or about forty grams per meal).

- **Total grams of low glycemic load carbohydrates per day** (process goal: 100 grams of carbs per day or less, or fifteen to twenty-five grams of carbs per meal).

- **Capsules of molecularly distilled fish oil** (process goal: 6–12 capsules per day depending upon her inflammation markers).

- **Minutes of full-body aerobic exercise per day** (process goal: at least 30 minutes, three times a week; 45 minutes, four to five times a week is even better).

- **Hours of sleep each night** (process goal: at least seven hours).

- **Supplements** (process goal: as defined in the Supplementation chapter).

- **Measurements** (process goal: her weight, waist measurement, and her navel and thigh skinfold measurements).

A third kind of goal completes her goal-setting process: performance goals. How does our average American woman know if she is actually making any progress toward her outcome goal of her ideal body weight at 22 percent body fat?

Performance goals let you know if you are moving in the right direction. The four most important performance goals to track daily are:

- **Weight** (performance goal of slow, steady weight loss averaging about one-half to no more than one pound per week).

- **Waist** (performance goal of slow, steady loss of inches around waist).

- **Navel Skinfold** (performance goal of slow, steady decrease in skinfold thickness, averaging about one-half millimeter per week).

- **Thigh Skinfold** (performance goal of slow, steady decrease in skinfold thickness averaging about one-half millimeter per week).

Once a week, do the full seven sites with your skinfold caliper, enter all your data into our website, and print your results. Create a binder, and build a history of your progress. These weekly body compositions tests will give you invaluable feedback as to your fat loss (or lack thereof), your muscle gain (or loss), and your rate of progress (or lack thereof). Your weekly body composition tests will also confirm that you are being dedicated enough to achieve your ultimate goal. If you are not progressing at the rate you thought you would, you need to bear down on your process goals each day. By consistently achieving your process goals every day (water, protein, exercise, sleep, etc.), you will ensure that you will make steady, measurable progress. In the chapter, "Listen to YOUR Body," we will explain exactly how to interpret your seven-site body composition results and how to adjust your daily process accordingly.

In the next chapter, "Control YOUR Environment," we will show you how to integrate your process goals with your environment, and we will underscore how critical it is to align your environment with your goals so you avoid mixed messages and eliminate the distractions and triggers from your environment that undermine your progress and your ultimate success. If you want a high-quality life, you must create a high-quality environment.

You can't build muscle with junk food.

Chapter 16

Control YOUR Environment

Keep your house clean, because if it is in your house, you (and your family) will eat it.

—Joe Dillon

When it comes to goals, the key question is: Does what I am about to do move me closer to my goal or not? If your answer is no, then don't do it. It is that simple. When you create your environment, this is the key question you need to ask yourself over and over again. As an example, does stocking your house with your favorite snack foods move you closer to your outcome goal of attaining your ideal weight or not? The answer is clearly no.

Does your environment align with your goal(s)? Or are you creating a mixed message? If you have something in your house that you know you just can't stop eating, you have a self-defeating mismatch between your environment and your goal. And remember, people are a powerful component of your environment. Therefore, a second big question becomes: Are the people in your life supportive of you and your goals, or do they sabotage you?

Creating an environment that is conducive to getting lean and optimally healthy is not a one-time thing. You will continue to fine-tune your environment as part of your ongoing process. As you learn more about health, as you learn about yourself and your weak spots, as you learn more about what actually helps you and what hurts you, you will continue to tweak your environment. Part of creating an environment that is conducive to accomplishing your goals is removing temptations. Also, part of creating an environment conducive to accomplishing your goals is making sure the tools and components you need are readily available.

As I said, if it is in your house, you WILL eat it. If you are committed to achieving and sustaining your goal of your ideal body weight, you need to continually pay attention to your environment. Does something (a certain food or drink) call out to you? Do you find yourself obsessing about a certain food or drink? When you do, eliminate it from your house. For whatever reason, you are addicted to this food or drink. If you are addicted, you can't even take one bite or it will set you off. If an alcoholic is serious about staying sober, he can't even take one single drink. He can't have alcohol of any kind in his house. He is powerless over this substance.

Your environment starts with where you live. This is the place over which you have the most control. The first step is to get your house squeaky clean, and eliminate anything that is not on your four lists (please see the Resource chapter for copies of all four lists, or visit our website, where members can download all the lists in this book). The next step is to stock up your house with plenty of water; several kinds of lean, complete proteins, especially whey protein isolate powder for your protein shakes and boneless, skinless chicken breasts; several kinds of low glycemic load carbohydrates such as leafy green vegetables like spinach, fresh or frozen vegetables like asparagus or broccoli, whole, fresh fruit such as apples and oranges, and frozen, unsweetened fruit like strawberries and blueberries; and some healthy fat, especially molecularly distilled fish oil capsules and some raw tree nuts like raw almonds.

In addition to pure water, healthy foods, and high-quality supplements, you will need healthy tools. These healthy tools should include such things as an accurate scale to measure your body weight, a skinfold caliper to measure your body fat, a tape measure to measure your waist, a blender to make your whey protein shakes, a heart rate monitor to measure your training heart rate, comfortable walking shoes, workout clothes, and light hand-weights.

Next, build an environment that constantly reminds you of your goals and of your new, healthier way of life. Have your blender out in plain sight on your kitchen counter. Your blender is a symbol of your commitment to a consistent intake of the eight essential amino acids your body requires to build muscle, keep your blood sugar stable, and support optimal health. Place a jar of whey protein isolate protein powder out in plain sight on your kitchen counter. Be sure it is pure whey protein isolate with no soy protein or casein protein added—and no added sugars or artificial sweeteners of any kind. You want to keep appetite stimulants out of your house. Artificial sweeteners increase your appetite and make you fat.

Staying well hydrated is fundamental to getting lean. Place bottles of water out in plain sight on your kitchen counter and within arm's reach at all times.

Keep your refrigerator stocked with cooked boneless, skinless chicken breasts. Cooked chicken breasts are a versatile lean protein. You can eat them cold, in a salad, or pop them in your microwave for thirty to sixty seconds and eat them hot. Cooked chicken travels well in your car, on the golf course, or on a plane.

Keep one or more bottles of supplements, especially molecularly distilled fish oil capsules, out in plain sight to remind you to take your six to twelve capsules every day.

Keep your scale in a prominent place so you see it often.

Keep your daily log out and open to your current day.

Pay attention to where and how you eat your meals at home. Beware of open containers. Big bowls of food served family style encourage overeating. Staring at all that food throughout your entire meal is a powerful appetite stimulant. Serve only what you plan to eat on a plate in your kitchen, then put the rest of the food away out of sight in the refrigerator. You can use smaller plates to help control your portions.

Part of getting leaner and healthier is self-responsibility and self-regulation. You have to take full responsibility for your body, your health, and the shape you are in. Part of losing weight (body fat) and getting leaner is accepting your own weaknesses. If you were a tower of strength, you would already be lean and fit. If that is not the case, you obviously have some work to do. Part of that work is learning how to protect yourself. And protecting yourself starts with your home. Your home should be your safe haven, a place where you can relax and feel safe without distractions or temptations.

You don't have to be perfect. Most people find it difficult to maintain this level of strictness 24/7, and Sandy and I are no exception. This is why we encourage you to have one to three treat meals per week. Feel free to experiment and try any foods you like, as well as those favorites you may be missing. Since you *do* get to indulge occasionally, this gives you something to look forward to and also allows you to integrate social events and "date nights" into your routine, without guilt.

The key is to tightly circumscribe your vices. Plan for when and where you will choose to have your treat meals. By planning ahead and making this choice a conscious decision, you are the one in control, and you will prevent yourself from falling into the trap of peer pressure and surprise derailments. By staying focused on *your* goals and listening to *your* body, you will find the right mix for *you*. But remember, keep your house clean. When you do indulge in treat meals, eat all of your treat meals outside your home, in a restaurant, or at a friend's home. Remember, home should be your safe haven, and only the items on our lists should be in your home.

At first, you may go crazy on your treat meals. But you will find over time that your treat meals slowly get cleaner. The leaner and healthier you get, the less appealing junk food becomes. As you get leaner and healthier, being hung over from binge eating or alcohol just won't make sense anymore.

Once you get your house clean and begin to live a healthier lifestyle, the next step is to extend your control to your other environments, starting with your car. First and foremost, stock your car up with water, including at least two six-packs of bottled water. And keep your car stocked up. You might carry a Ziploc bag of raw almonds in your car. Raw almonds will stay fairly fresh in a Ziploc bag. Raw almonds are a good fallback if you get caught out and find yourself hungry. With water and raw almonds, you will be just fine. As you get more sophisticated, you can carry a cooler in your car. Carry a towel in your car to keep your clothes clean. If you spend a lot of time in your car doing outside sales, for example, you should get yourself a good hard-shell cooler and stock it up every day before you leave home. Your cooler should always contain the basics: cold water, chicken breasts, and some easy-to-eat fresh fruit like apples or sliced raw vegetables. Even better, make a couple of protein shakes and carry them in Nalgene bottles. With shakes, chicken, water, fruit, vegetables, and raw almonds, you are set for a full, productive day.

Many people go to an office to work. Create a lean, healthy environment in your car for your drive to and from your office. This is especially important if you have a commute of an hour or more each way to work. Bring a soft cooler with your lunch and snacks to support your process goals throughout your workday. When you bring your food from home, you will eat cleaner and healthier; and you will also save money, and save time previously spent going out to lunch to eat a less-than-healthy meal. If you eat a clean, high-protein lunch, you will be amazed how much more energetic and productive you will be in the afternoon.

If you travel more extensively, as I do, then you know airports and airplanes are very challenging environments. As I shared, I have been flying one hundred thousand to two hundred thousand miles a year for decades. For me, a small, soft, portable cooler is an essential travel tool. I can bring a one-liter Nalgene bottle with two scoops of my protein powder already in it. Once through security, I buy some bottles of water. I add sixteen to twenty-four ounces of cold water to my Nalgene bottle, shake it a few times, and I have a great tasting drink containing forty-eight to fifty grams of perfect protein. I take my supplements with my shake. Then I eat an apple and ten to twelve raw almonds to complete my clean, balanced meal. I carry extra travel packs of protein powder for meals later in the day. A one-liter Nalgene bottle, some travel packs of whey protein isolate (each pack is two scoops of whey protein isolate), a couple of apples, a small Ziploc baggie of raw almonds, and your supplements, and you are good to go. It is easy to get a couple more apples in any airport. And you can buy bottled water in any airport. I find small bags of raw almonds at most newsstands. If you eat a healthy meal *before* your flight, you won't be tempted by the alcohol or junk food on the plane. Carry at least one full sixteen- to twenty-four-ounce bottle of water on each domestic flight, and much more for longer international flights.

Your biggest single challenge when you fly will be dehydration. The inside of an airplane, which is bone dry and pressurized at about eight thousand feet altitude, is an extremely dehydrating environment. You need to make sure you bring enough water. You can never count on the flight attendants to provide you with enough water. Also, you need to avoid anything that dehydrates you, such as alcohol of any kind, sodas of any kind, candy, or salty snacks. Remember: You are the only person who actually cares about your health. The airline certainly does not. Be prepared to drink at least eight ounces of water for every hour you are on the plane. This is the number one reason I always get an aisle seat.

If you do get caught out at an airport and you have no food, do not despair. You can get grilled chicken breasts at virtually any fast-food restaurant. Virtually all fast-food restaurants sell some kind of a grilled (not fried) chicken sandwich. Lose the bread. Just order your chicken breasts a la carte. Get a dinner salad with Italian dressing or an apple, plus a bottle of water, and you are set.

In every environment or situation you find yourself, the key questions are: What is the reality of my current situation? And given that reality, what are my healthiest alternatives? Think your situation through and respond. Be proactive, rather than reactive. Our obesogenic culture has built knee-jerk reactions into all of us. You need to keep your head, use your brain, and make rational decisions. You want to live on purpose, based upon your values and your goals. You are not some helpless mouse trapped in a maze. You have more control over your environment and your responses than you may realize. And when your environment is less controllable, you can still make reasonably healthy choices. In my travels, I hear too many people say: "I am stuck at the airport; there is nothing I can do." They play the victim, disempower themselves, then crash and burn food-wise. Don't surrender your control. There is always a healthier choice. Of course, the most effective choice is to be prepared.

Another valuable tip is to avoid letting yourself get overly hungry and/or overly tired. When you are overly hungry and/or tired, you are much more vulnerable in any situation or environment. When you get overly tired, you tend to regress to old, neurotic, self-destructive behaviors. This is one reason business travel is such a challenge. Often due to circumstances beyond your control (a cancelled flight, for instance), you may end up stuck at an airport, bored and tired. You're better off getting the healthiest thing you can to eat and drink (you can always get bottled water and raw almonds), and then taking a nap.

Once you get to your destination city and pick up your rental car, your best bet is to head for a market near your hotel. I always map out a grocery store near my hotel. I always stay at a hotel with a kitchen, including at least a full refrigerator and microwave. I always check the store hours ahead of time to be sure it will be open when I land, even if I get in late. Many markets are open twenty-four hours a day. Be prepared with a grocery list. Don't fall into the trap of winging it when you are tired and hungry. At the top of your list, of course, is water. I buy a six pack of twenty-four-ounce bottles of water for each day I will be in a city. Apples and raw almonds are next on my list. You can always find raw almonds in the baking section of any supermarket and/or in the produce section. With the basics of water, raw almonds, and apples, you will always be in good shape, particularly if you carry travel packs of whey protein isolate powder and a one-liter Nalgene bottle.

It may not be fancy or exciting, but it is super healthy. If it is early enough in the evening when you get to the market, they may have a salad bar. Salad bars are double-edged swords. You can eat really healthily, or you can get into real trouble. Optimally, you are not overly hungry. If you land hungry, get some raw almonds and eat a handful to take the edge off your hunger.

With salad bars, your basic formula is simple: a bed of greens like spinach and/or Romaine lettuce, some lean, complete protein like chicken or turkey or hard boiled eggs, then topped with a thin dressing like oil and vinegar or Italian. Avoid the heavy, creamy dressings. To add more protein to your meal and/or to "beef-up" your salad, you might get a roasted chicken. These are typically not perfect, but you can get some first-class protein. They are usually a little salty. Avoid the skin, which is pure fat. But feel free to eat the rest. If you are going to be in this town for a couple of days, prepare several salads of greens. Keep them in the refrigerator in your hotel room. Pick up a bottle of olive oil and vinegar or olive oil–based Italian dressing. You can then use the meat from your roasted chicken to provide your lean protein for several nearly perfect meals.

Your hotel room is your home away from home. Rule number one: Keep your house (on the road) clean. Don't use being on the road as an excuse to blow your eating plan. Only bring water and foods on your four lists into your room. Never bring alcohol into your room. Or junk food. Control your TV time. Instead, take advantage of your time on the road to get more sleep and catch up on your reading. Use the quiet time to think, plan, and be productive. Your first priority is sleep. Be your own best friend. Don't you be the cause of exhaustion, if you can help it. Time on the road is work time. It's time to focus on your job and on your health. The better shape you are in, the more effective you will be at your work.

Business meetings, whether in your hometown or on the road, are fraught with potential pitfalls. Alcohol is a big one. You will do your best work sober. You will get more done and close more deals if your brain is clear and well-rested. Getting sloshed on the road is going to put you in a big hole from which you will not recover the rest of your trip. Avoid going to a business lunch or dinner starved. If you arrive overly hungry, you are going to be vulnerable to all the temptations. Remember: Alcohol lowers your inhibitions. Also, alcohol relaxes your smooth muscles, meaning that you can overeat and not realize how full you really are. You can do a lot of damage with a combination of alcohol and tempting food. If you are prepared, you can choose consciously and selectively, minimizing the damage in even the worst of circumstances. Carry some raw almonds to take the edge off your appetite and bolster your will power. Also, if you know you have food back at your hotel room, you will not be quite so desperate at the meeting.

One of the toughest challenges at business meetings is peer pressure. Your business colleagues may not be as emotionally mature as you or as serious about their career as you, so you have to protect yourself. Don't sell your soul just to be one of the boys (or girls). This is your career. This is your job. Being super smart and high-energy all the time are two crucial components of success at anything you do. You control how clear and sharp your brain is and how much energy you have. Avoid squandering opportunities. We only get so many opportunities in life. Success is often not about how many opportunities you get, but what you do with the opportunities presented to you. Keep yourself in position to take full advantage of every opportunity that life presents to you. This is how you do your best. It's like the old joke: Opportunity knocked, but I didn't hear it because I had the TV on.

Social environments are different from business environments. In business, the key is to keep your eye on the ball at all times. As a result, to be fully productive and effective, you want to be clean and sober. Going into a social environment, you need to ask yourself one key question before you go: Is this going to be one of my treat meals for the week, or am I going to try to stick to my clean, healthy eating plan? If you plan to stick to your eating plan, eat ahead of time so you are not overly hungry and make sure you are fully hydrated before you go. But if this social situation will count as one of your treat meals, then anything goes. Go enjoy yourself guilt-free. Just never drink and drive.

You only get one life. You only get so much time. Your time is finite. There is an absolute end. Here's a fundamental question: How are you going to spend your time? You are in control of your time and your environment. No one else is looking out for you or your health. That is *your* job.

We live in an obesogenic environment where there are an infinite number of food and drink temptations. You will also often find yourself surrounded by those who will attempt to sabotage your efforts by pushing temptations on you. Stay strong and focused. Fat is contagious. Fat friends make us fat. And (the body does not lie) clearly, most Americans don't care about their health or the health of their children. So choose your partner and your friends well. Getting and staying lean and healthy has never been more challenging. Health is a value. What do you *really* value? If you really value your health, then your body will reflect it. Your body does not lie. As Gandhi said, "My life is my message." Create environments (including the people) that are consistent with *your* goals and *your* values.

Chapter 17

Control YOUR Day

Refine your process constantly and forever.
—Joe Dillon (an homage to
W. Edwards Deming, the father of quality)

You can see the step-by-step progression. First, you establish your goals: your outcome goal (such as attaining and maintaining your ideal body weight), your process goals (such as daily water intake, daily protein intake, etc.), and your performance goals (such as weight, waist, navel and thigh skinfold measurements). Next, you create an environment (including the people in your life) that is consistent with and supports your goals. The third step covered in this chapter is to create your day. Through conscious, deliberate thought; through trial and error; through daily and weekly measurements; through analysis, and through constant fine-tuning and course corrections, you create *your* optimal twenty-four-hour day. Your twenty-four-hour day is *your* process. Your day is a process that you will refine constantly and forever.

I have admired, studied, and have been around world-class athletes most of my life. I learned early on that many of the great ones had very particular and involved daily routines that helped them consistently produce outstanding performances and achieve excellence. One of the athletes I most respect and admire is Raymond Berry. Berry was not a guy you would have ever picked to become one of the greatest receivers of all time. Berry had a number of challenges: one leg was slightly shorter than the other; he had to wear contact lenses; he was not fast; he was not strong. He was not a superstar in either high school or college. But Berry was a thinker, an analyzer, and a goal-setter. And Berry was dedicated to his goals.

Raymond Berry's professional football career began inauspiciously. He was drafted in the twentieth round. He barely made the Baltimore Colts. But he immediately began to build his process. He borrowed a projector and studied game films. This was in the mid-1950s, long before watching game films was a standard practice. Berry was looking for any edge to help him overcome his challenges. Watching other receivers, he noticed a good fake could compensate for lack of speed. Berry worked diligently and developed a huge repertoire of fakes. Berry got so good at fakes that he could get open against even the best defenders. He lifted weights. Again, this was way before weight training became a standard practice. He realized that his hands were his greatest asset, so he constantly squeezed Silly Putty to strengthen his fingers. Most players arrived at camp out of shape and played themselves into shape. From his second camp on, Berry arrived in superb condition on day one of camp and was always in superb condition.

Raymond Berry discovered early on, through trial and error and paying close attention, that he played his best at a certain weight. For his entire thirteen-year pro career, Berry kept his weight within one pound of his ideal playing weight. How did he manage to do this? Berry developed a daily process. He weighed himself every single morning (at home or on the road) and wrote it down. Controlling his environment, Berry carried the same bathroom scale wherever he went—even in his suitcase for road games. If he weighed less than his optimal playing weight that morning, he would eat slightly more food that day. But if he weighed more than his optimal playing weight, he would eat slightly less food that day.

Berry had a clearly defined performance goal: precisely maintain his optimal playing weight. Based on his goal, he controlled his environments and his daily process. He took control of his environment and carried his own scale. First, he was not at the mercy of the hotel whether he had a scale or not. And second, he always used exactly the same scale so his daily process would not be thrown off by different scales.

How successful was Raymond Berry's daily process? Berry became a Pro Football Hall of Fame wide receiver for the Baltimore Colts and played on two World Championship teams. Berry was a multi-time All-Pro. But for me, two of his most remarkable statistics: in thirteen years as a professional football player, he dropped a total of two passes and only fumbled once.

Berry had seemingly insurmountable challenges. But Berry set his goals. He became famous for his preparation and attention to detail. He made sure he had the tools to support his pursuit of his goals, such as his projector, weights, Silly Putty, and his bathroom scale. The point: Accomplishing your goals is *not* an accident or luck. Setting and accomplishing your goals is a conscious, deliberate, methodical, day-to-day process. Adjust your process based on objective feedback (in Berry's case, his weight every morning on his scale).

Based on your goals and your temperament, let's construct an optimal day. The idea is to work your day, every day, retaining those elements that clearly support your goals and your success, and eliminating those elements that clearly block or interfere with your goals. The result: Over time, you will build the most effective process to attain and maintain your goals.

Given the challenges we all face, what actions can you take and what behaviors can you implement that help you effectively lose weight?

Your day really starts the night before when you go to bed and turn the lights out. Why? Because letting yourself get exhausted will make you fat. Getting a sound night's sleep of at least seven hours is essential to having an effective day. So one of the first process goals for you to establish is: What is the optimal time for you to get into bed, turn out the lights, and get to sleep?

Your next process goal is: What is the optimal time (approximately) for you to get up, given that one of your performance goals is getting at least seven hours of sound sleep each night?

When you wake up in the morning, record in your daily log the time you turned off the lights last night; the time you woke up; and the total number of hours of sound sleep you got. Then go to the bathroom. Strip down and start your morning measurement routine. Weigh yourself and write down your actual weight in pounds. Measure your waist at the navel with a tape measure. Stand relaxed. Don't suck it in. Pull your tape just until it is taut. Record the circumference of your waist in inches. Measure the thickness of your navel skinfold one inch from the center of your navel with your skinfold caliper. Grab a vertical skinfold and pull the fold of your skin and subcutaneous fat away from your abdominal muscles. Record the thickness of your navel skinfold in millimeters. Measure the thickness of your thigh skinfold midway between your hip and your kneecap, grabbing a vertical fold of skin. Record your thigh skinfold.

Essential tools for your process: binder, daily logs, pen, scale, skinfold caliper, and measuring tape.

Breakfast is one of the most important meals, if not *the* most important meal of your day. If you are not a morning exerciser, a shake is a perfect meal for breakfast. Into your blender pour sixteen ounces of water or nonfat milk, two level scoops of whey protein isolate, and one medium piece of whole, fresh fruit or up to one cup of frozen, unsweetened fruit. Put the top on and blend. If you want your shake thicker and/or colder, you can add ice. If you use both ice and frozen, unsweetened fruit, you will end up with a very thick shake. Drink your shake with your morning supplements. Although a shake is an ideal breakfast, you may decide you would prefer a different choice. Perhaps an egg white omelet (remember to include enough protein in your omelet. That means you need about 1.5–2 cups of egg whites) with vegetables. Record this meal in your daily log.

If you prefer to workout first thing in the morning, you still need to eat. However, the next step in your process is to get *half* a shake into your body before your morning workout. Why? To protect your lean body mass. Make a half shake composed of eight to ten ounces of water or nonfat milk, one scoop of whey protein isolate, and half a piece of fruit. Blend and drink. Record this in your daily log. If you are concerned about waking your family with the noise of your blender, make your half shake the night before. Store your half shake in a half-liter or liter Nalgene bottle. Then, in the morning, all you have to do is give the Nalgene bottle a couple of quick shakes, drink, and you are set.

Essential tools for this part of your process: blender, water or nonfat milk, jar of natural whey protein isolate, whole, fresh fruit like bananas or frozen, unsweetened fruit like frozen blueberries, shake cup, half-liter or one-liter Nalgene bottle.

Put on your workout gear. Be sure to wear a chest-strap heart rate monitor to keep track of your training heart rate. Grab your light hand-weights and go for your thirty to forty-five minute walk.

Immediately upon your return, record your workout in your daily log (depending on the model of your chest-strap heart rate monitor): total time, average training heart rate, maximum heart rate, recovery heart rate, calories burned, weight of hand-weights, and repetitions per set. Then drink a full protein shake to kick-start your recovery process and take full advantage of your three-hour anabolic window. This shake should include sixteen ounces of water or nonfat milk, two level scoops of whey protein isolate, and one medium piece of whole, fresh fruit or up to one cup of frozen, unsweetened fruit. If you want your recovery shake thicker and/ or colder, you can add ice. Drink your recovery shake with your morning supplements. Record in your daily log.

By the way, any time you use water to make your shakes, that water counts toward your 8 to 12, eight-ounce glasses of pure water per day.

Shower, dress, and get ready for work or the rest of your day.

Next, think through your food for the rest of your day. To take full advantage of your three-hour anabolic window, be prepared to eat a second meal before your three-hour window closes. With each meal or shake, you are trying to find the optimal pattern (the most effective combination of lean proteins, slow-burning carbs, and healthy fats) that works for you. Once you find a meal or shake that works for you, record a clear definition of that meal or shake.

From that point on, keep your meal or shake as close to uniform as you can. When you find something that is effective, don't change it. Build your daily process on a foundation of proven, effective blocks. Soon you will have a solid edifice of proven, effective behaviors that will carry you to your goal and beyond. Plan your day by packing your cooler with water, premade shakes, cooked chicken breasts, whole, fresh fruit, raw almonds, etc.

Essential tools to eat healthily and thrive in an obesogenic environment: soft or hard shell cooler; Blue Ice to keep your water, shakes, and food cold; bottles of water; precooked chicken breasts, whole, fresh fruit, and a stock of raw almonds.

If you have exercised, eat a midmorning meal as the second meal in your three-hour anabolic window. If you have not exercised in the morning, you will need a midmorning meal as well. This might be another shake. Or it might be a chicken breast, an apple, and ten to twelve raw almonds.

Lunch is where many people begin to blow their day. If people at work go out to lunch, they waste an enormous amount of time, energy, and money, and most of the time, they end up eating something that compromises their weight-loss goal as well as their productive energy for the afternoon. In addition, if you go out with coworkers, you leave yourself open to peer pressure. Keep in mind (look around, the body does not lie) that most people do not care about their health. If you are eating lunch with a bunch of people who don't care about their health, there is going to be tremendous pressure to eat where they want to eat (such as a pizza place or pasta place or fast-food) and your choices to eat healthy and stay on track to accomplish your goals will be either severely limited or nonexistent.

It is a sad but true fact: If you are going to get and stay lean, you are going to have to look out for yourself. Don't expect any help from friends or coworkers. In fact, expect constant attempts to undermine your healthy efforts. The weak always try to tear down the strong. You are either going to have to be very strong-willed and assert yourself, or you are going to have to change your lunch-time social habits. In either case, expect to get major grief. It's a lot more fun to eat pizza and drink soft drinks for lunch than it is to eat a lean, healthy meal. But if you stick to your guns, you will stay on track to accomplish your health goals (ideal body weight, etc.), and you will have dramatically more energy in the afternoon. Eat a clean, healthy meal with plenty of pure water, and you will be significantly more productive in the afternoon. You will be wide-awake and in a positive, upbeat mood all afternoon. By sticking with your eating plan, you will not only move closer to your ideal body weight, you will also be more successful in your job. A healthy meal at this time might be another shake. Or it might be a can of water-packed tuna on a bed of greens with a little olive oil and balsamic vinegar, or a chicken breast, an apple, and ten to twelve raw almonds.

Next, be prepared to eat a small, clean, balanced meal midway through your afternoon. This meal will keep your blood sugar stable, your mind clear, your energy up, and keep you on track to accomplish your goal of attaining your ideal body weight. Your midafternoon meal will also sustain your stable blood sugar for another three to five hours so you don't arrive home for dinner starved. If you prefer to work out in the later afternoon or early evening, after work, then a midafternoon meal is essential. Again, at this time, the concepts for this meal remain the same as your previous meals. However, if you are going to be working out within forty-five minutes to one hour of this meal, a two-scoop shake will be your best choice.

If you need to shop for food on the way home, your midafternoon meal is even more important. If, as you leave work, you feel a little hungry, eat a small handful of raw almonds and drink eight to sixteen ounces of water to take the edge off your hunger. Never shop hungry, and *always* shop with a list. Only buy what is on your list. No impulse buys allowed. Remember, if you buy it, you *will* eat it. When you buy chicken, don't buy one or two breasts. Buy five or ten pounds of boneless, skinless chicken breasts.

If you arrive home with the intention of working out before dinner, make sure you keep this appointment with yourself. Don't settle into the easy chair and turn on the TV. Keep moving right through your house, change your clothes, put on your chest-strap monitor and your workout gear, and get out the door. Don't lose your momentum. Especially if you feel tired. It is counterintuitive, but your workout will actually energize you. Why? When you walk with light hand-weights, you are significantly speeding up your metabolism and cranking more oxygen through your body and, especially, your brain. You will return from your 30 to 45 minute walk with light hand-weights wide awake and refreshed. It is like a fresh start to your day.

Drink a full recovery shake immediately upon completing your workout. Record your workout in your daily log as you drink your shake. Preheat your oven to 375 degrees. Enjoy your shower. You have earned it.

After your shower, bake your chicken in your preheated oven. Five pounds of boneless, skinless chicken breasts will cover the bottom of one broiler pan. Bake your chicken for exactly twenty-five minutes with a timer. Do not leave cooking to chance. While your chicken is cooking, you could make a tossed green salad. Remember, you can eat unlimited leafy green vegetables. Leafy green vegetables are the healthiest carbohydrates you can eat. You can also include vegetables, such as a variety of bell peppers (green, red, yellow, orange) and grape tomatoes. Use raw organic flax seed oil or extra virgin olive oil plus balsamic vinegar for your dressing.

One or two medium-sized chicken breasts with a big tossed-green salad is an incredibly healthy meal for you and your family. Drink lots of water with your meal.

Here are some additional healthy ideas to add taste and interest to your chicken, turkey, fish or game meat: salsa, mustard, salt-free seasonings, garlic powder, onion powder, tarragon, basil, dill, and/or any spices and herbs that you like. Feel free to experiment with these to find the ones you enjoy the most.

Quite often, people ask us for recipes, but the key to really being successful is to keep things simple and easy. Gone are the excuses that cooking at home just takes too much time and that you are too busy to eat healthy. Don't complicate things with elaborate recipes. No recipes are needed when you are eating clean, healthy meals. Besides, food in its pure form actually tastes better.

Record your dinner in your daily log.

If sleep is an issue for you, taking one 3 mg capsule of sustained-release melatonin will help. Follow your usual meal template for your presleep meal: a fist of lean, complete protein; plus a fist or a cup of slow-burning, low glycemic load carbohydrates; plus a thumb of raw, healthy fat like ten to twelve raw almonds. This could be one medium-sized chicken breast, one medium-sized apple, and ten to twelve raw almonds, or an egg white omelet with one and a half to two cups of egg whites, avocado, and some spinach. If your dinner is within sixty to ninety minutes of your bedtime, you may not need a presleep meal.

Next, brush and floss your teeth. Make sure you have an environment that is conducive to a sound night's sleep: cool (sixty-five degrees is optimal), dark (pitch black is optimal), and quiet (the quieter, the better). Get in bed. Read a book. When you feel the first wave of drowsiness, close your book, turn off your light, and settle down to go to sleep.

This is your baseline pattern.

Since incorporating treat meals into your routine is also part of your lifestyle, an integral part to long-term success is not only planning your optimal *day*, but also your optimal *week*.

Business and/or vacation travel will multiply your challenges. Stay focused on your outcome goal (attaining your ideal body weight). You will make mistakes. We will address setbacks in the chapter, "Manage YOUR Setbacks."

Avoid wasting valuable psychic energy beating yourself up if and when you do slip. Instead, use your limited energy resources to learn and modify your pattern to lessen the likelihood of making the same slip-up again. Trial and error. Live and learn. This is *your* process. By consistently recording and analyzing, you can distill your lessons into a lifestyle that reflects your schedule and your temperament. With conscious, concerted, methodical effort, your process will soon fit you like a glove. As your tailor-made process begins to produce tangible, empirical results (lowering of skinfolds, lowering of body fat, and increase in your lean body mass), you will realize that if you adhere to your process, you will never have excess body fat again. You will have reclaimed *your* body and *your* life.

Chapter 18

Listen to YOUR Body

YOUR body does not lie.
—Author unknown

The goal of life is to be healthy and happy, to build a life to rejoice in, a life of fulfillment and meaning and value, to contribute. This is true health. Health is foundational to happiness because it is pretty hard to be happy if you are sick, especially if you are seriously sick. Your job is to learn to pay attention to what makes you healthy and happy and do more of that; to notice what makes you unhealthy and/or unhappy, and do your best to eliminate these behaviors; to rise above the empty, superficial, aimless, and flailing around of popular culture and mass media. To discover who YOU are and what YOU want. Your job is to learn how to build your health, to build meaningful relationships, which are so much a part of true happiness, and to build wealth (financial security), so you are less buffeted by the vagaries of the market.

To do this, you need to expand your time frame from instant gratification (emotional immaturity) to delayed gratification (adult, mature, healthier emotional state). For example, when we are young, it may be fun to get drunk. But having a bad night and waking up hung over with a headache and feeling nauseous—is the cost really worth the benefit? As you get older and have more responsibilities, you can't afford to lose a couple of days feeling bad, irritable, and unproductive. Even in college, if you want to do well (e.g., get good grades and actually get an education), you can't afford to waste too much time drinking and partying versus studying and getting your rest so you can learn most effectively. Even in high school and college, we have goals, whether that is to excel at sports and/or academics.

The basic process to getting healthy is to first establish a baseline. Once you ascertain where you are, then you set a goal or goals. Next, you formulate a plan: How do you intend to accomplish your goal? Then you begin to act or behave. You measure the results of your behaviors. You evaluate which behaviors moved you closer to your goals (constructive) and which behaviors moved you away from your goals (self-destructive). Then, based on those lessons, you modify your behaviors and act again. This is a never-ending process meant to increase the amount of time you are healthy and happy and accomplishing *your* goals and decreasing the amount of time you feel lost, lonely, depressed, or sick. Your process will never give you 100 percent health and happiness, but with consistent effort, you can build a life in which the majority of time you are truly healthy and sincerely happy. That is as good as it gets. Learn to be thankful for that.

Your whole process begins with listening to your body. What does it mean *to listen* to your body? To listen means to pay attention to your body, to look at your body, to observe your body, and to measure your body. Your body does not lie. Your body will always give you accurate feedback. Your body will tell you whether you are thriving, surviving, or struggling. A major key to your process is to get in touch, and stay in touch, with the empirical reality of your body.

In this chapter, you will learn what to pay attention to and what your perceptions mean. You will learn to pay attention to your skin, your urine, your stomach, your skinfolds, and your blood—to name just a few invaluable sources of information. Every aspect of your body has a wealth of information about the status of your health and how your health (physical, mental, and emotional) is affecting your mood.

Whenever you eat a meal, pay attention to how you feel at the start of your meal. How hungry are you? Did you let yourself get overly hungry? Letting yourself get overly hungry is asking for trouble. Small to moderate meals eaten more frequently is a more effective eating strategy. As you eat, pay attention to when you no longer feel hungry. Not full. Just no longer hungry. This is when you should stop eating. Eating until you are full is too much food. And if you eat until you are full on a consistent basis, you will get fat.

Your goal is to keep yourself between neutral and satisfied. Try to avoid getting ravenously hungry. The hungrier you get, the longer it takes for a feeling of satiety to kick in to stop you from eating. By the same token, try to avoid stuffing yourself. Eating until you feel full often leads to overeating because by the time you feel full, you have eaten way too much food. A half-hour later, you will be beyond full. You are stuffed. Listen to your body.

Try to determine the combination of foods (lean proteins, etc.) and the amounts of these foods that satisfy your hunger, but allow you to still feel good a half-hour or so after the meal. Pay attention to how long it takes for your feeling of satiety to kick in. Your body may have a slow sense of satiety, in which case you have to learn to stop eating before you feel satisfied, knowing that a half-hour or forty-five minutes later, you will feel just right. This is where pre-planned meals or uniform meals come in. You may be one of those people who can only eat half of what you want to eat, because if you eat all that you want to eat at any given meal, a half-hour later you will realize you have totally overeaten and you'll feel stuffed and uncomfortable. Some of you may have to constantly monitor your eating—what you eat, when you eat, and your portion size—in order to eat in such a way that you can get and stay lean. This is your personal challenge.

Water is a good place to start. Water is crucial to your health and to losing weight. How do you know if you are well hydrated? Thirst is one indication. Unfortunately, by the time you experience thirst, you are well on your way to dehydration. As you get older, thirst becomes an even less reliable indicator of your level of hydration. The color of your urine is a much more reliable indicator of your hydration level. Optimal hydration is indicated by nearly clear urine or urine that is a slight straw color. As your urine takes on a darker color, you are becoming dehydrated. Dark yellow means you are dehydrated. A brownish color indicates an even more advanced state of dehydration. Taking large amounts of supplements can complicate your urine signal. For a few hours after you take a big batch of supplements, your urine will be darker yellow. But after a while, if you are well hydrated, your urine should become almost clear. The lesson? When you go to the bathroom, look at your urine. The color of your urine provides invaluable information about your hydration status.

Your heart rate is another signal rich in useful information. Your resting heart rate is one indication of your cardiovascular fitness level. Resting heart rate varies among people. As you get into an aerobic exercise program, your resting heart rate will begin to decrease. This is a reliable indicator that you are getting into better aerobic shape. For most people, a resting heart rate in the sixties is an indicator of *good* aerobic fitness. A resting heart rate in the fifties is an indicator of *very good* aerobic fitness. And a resting heart rate in the forties is an indicator of *excellent* aerobic fitness. The most important indicator is the trend of your resting heart rate. No matter where you start, if your resting heart rate gets lower over time (weeks and months) as you exercise aerobically, you are getting into better aerobic condition, meaning you are able to supply more oxygen to your body and to your brain.

You have an optimal training heart rate range. A simple and conservative formula is 220 minus your current age to determine your maximum heart rate. Then take 75 percent of your maximum heart rate to establish your upper limit. Take 60 percent of your maximum heart rate to determine your lower limit. You will get optimal improvement in your aerobic fitness if you keep your training heart rate within your optimal training heart rate range for at least thirty to forty-five minutes, at least three to five times each week. But again, if you pay attention, you will notice that as you get into better cardiovascular shape, you will have to worker harder just to get your training heart rate above 60 percent. This is a good sign. It means your heart is getting stronger and can do more work.

Another perspective on your aerobic fitness is your recovery heart rate. Recovery heart rate means how long it takes for your training heart rate to come back down to normal or close to your resting heart rate. The faster your heart recovers from your workout, the better shape you are in. Faster recovery means your heart is stronger and more resilient. The faster your recovery heart rate, the more energy you will have and the more effectively you will deal with stress.

In more extreme circumstances, a rising heart rate is an indicator of dehydration. As you become dehydrated, your heart rate will begin to accelerate both at rest and as you exercise. I have experienced this directly during a hike in the Grand Canyon when the temperature on the floor of the canyon was 110 degrees. The air was bone dry. I always wear my chest-strap heart rate monitor when I hike. As I began to get dehydrated, I could literally watch my heart rate begin to climb even though I was not walking any faster. Then, when I chugged a quart of water, I could watch my exercising heart rate settle back down into my optimal training heart rate range. Aron Ralston, the hiker whose right hand was pinned under an eight-hundred-pound boulder in a slot canyon in Utah for 127 hours, talks explicitly about this phenomenon in his book *Between A Rock and A Hard Place.*

Eight amino acids are essential to your health. How do you know if you are getting an optimal amount of lean, complete protein? One indicator is hunger. If you are eating an optimal amount of lean, complete protein with each of your four to six daily meals, you should experience little or no hunger. Why? Because an optimal amount of lean, complete protein with each meal will keep your blood sugar stable and prevent insulin spikes. This is also why we encourage you to measure your skinfolds every day: to measure the status of your lean body mass. If you are getting an optimal amount of lean, complete protein, your lean body mass will stay the same or slowly increase. If you are undereating lean, complete protein, you will experience constant hunger, and your lean body mass will slowly decline. Your body does not lie.

Other indicators of your intake of lean, complete protein include your nails and your hair. Your fingernails and hair are made out of protein. If you are eating optimal amounts of lean, complete protein, your fingernails will grow faster and be stronger and harder; your hair will grow faster and be healthier and stronger. Whoever cuts your hair may notice and remark on the health of your hair.

How about your carbohydrate intake? How will your body communicate with you about your carbohydrate intake? The first indicator of over-carbing is usually sleepiness. Eating more carbohydrates than *your* body can tolerate (people vary in their tolerance of sugar) will cause your blood sugar to spike. Any time you feel sleepy or drowsy after a meal, that is a pretty good indicator that you have exceeded your tolerance for sugar. The answer is to increase your intake of lean, complete protein and decrease your intake of carbohydrates (sugar). When you get to the ratio that is right for *your* body, you will feel no sleepiness after your meals. Instead, you will feel energized.

A less immediate indicator, but one that shows up pretty quickly, is an increase in your skinfold measurement. If you faithfully do your four measurements every morning and record them, you will soon notice how quickly your body responds to imbalances in your diet. If you begin to consistently over-carb, your skinfolds will increase within two to three days. That's how quickly you are beginning to get fatter. By the same to-ken, if you strictly adhere to a clean, well-balanced way of eating (a fist of lean, complete protein; plus a fist of slow-burning carbs; plus a thumb of raw, healthy fat), your skinfolds will begin to subtly decrease within two to three days.

What about your essential fat intake? The single most effective way to ensure that you are getting an optimal amount of essential fat (omega-3) is to take molecularly distilled fish oil capsules every day. The optimal range is six to twelve capsules per day. How do you know if you are get-ting enough fish oil? Dry skin is one good indicator, particularly on your heels and your elbows. When the skin of your heels and elbows is soft and pliable as opposed to being dry and cracked, you may be getting enough fish oil.

Painful joints are another indicator you are not getting enough fish oil (essential fat). When your skin and joints feel fluid and pliable, you may be getting enough fish oil. On the other hand, if your skin is red and cracked and psoriatic, or your joints hurt, you are not getting enough fish oil. How do you know if you may be getting too much fish oil for your body?   Es-sential fat is a crucial component for healthy bowels. But if you are taking twelve fish oil capsules a day and your bowels begin to get loose, twelve capsules a day may be too much for your body. Slowly and incrementally cut back from twelve to eleven. Wait a day or two to see if things settle down. If not, cut back from eleven to ten and so on, until you are where you want to be. By proceeding methodically and listening to *your* body, you can dial in the optimal dose of fish oil for your body.

What is YOUR body telling you with your four morning measurements?

- **Weight.** Dehydration can cause weight loss. Are you fully hydrated? Fluid retention can cause you to gain weight. Did you eat a salty meal or salty food? Did you over-carb? Every gram of carbohydrate retains four grams of water. No change in weight? What happened with your skinfolds? If your skinfold measurements improved (your skinfolds got smaller), but you did not lose weight, that means you gained muscle and lost fat. That is your goal. Weight by itself doesn't really tell you much. But if you combine your weight with your waist, navel, and thigh skinfold measurements, then you can begin to decipher what is going on with your body.

- **Waist.** Your waist measurement, like your weight, is a blunt instrument. If you simply eat less, your waist circumference may decrease. If you eat more, your waist circumference may increase. You are watching for trends. Is your weight trending downward? Is your waist circumference trending downward? To shed more light on your weight and waist measurements, you need to see the results of your skinfold measurements. If your weight remains constant or increases but your skinfolds decrease, you are getting leaner, increasing your lean body mass and decreasing your body fat. If you lose weight, your waist decreases, and your skinfolds decrease, this may be due to temporary dehydration. Make sure you are well hydrated. But if your skinfolds and your waist *continue* to trend downward, then you are getting leaner.

- **2 Skinfolds.** Navel and thigh. Your daily skinfold measurements will add real insight into your weight-loss process. Your skinfold calipers will tell you what kind of weight you are losing: fat or muscle. Remember, your goal is to lose fat and gain muscle.

To take your navel skinfold, flex your abdominal muscles. Dig your fingers in until you feel your abdominal muscles. With your dominant thumb and forefinger (most people are right-handed), grab a vertical fold of skin and pull your skin and fat away from your abdominal muscles. Hang on to your skinfold. With your other hand, place the tips of your skinfold calipers *behind* the fold. Take your finger off the trigger and let the gauge settle down until it stops. This is the thickness of your navel skinfold in millimeters. Write your actual skinfold measurement down.

To take your thigh skinfold: whichever thigh you are going to use, put your weight on the other thigh. With your dominant thumb and forefinger, grab a vertical fold of skin and fat midway between your hip and your knee cap. Pull your skinfold away from your thigh muscle. Place the tips of your skinfold caliper *behind* the fold. Take your finger off the trigger. Let the gauge settle down until it stops. This is the thickness of your thigh skinfold in millimeters. Write it down.

Do these four measurements every morning and watch the trends. The cleaner you eat, the more often you exercise, the more water your drink, and the more sleep you get, the faster your four measurements will decrease. Your body does not lie.

Establishing Your Baseline

At the beginning of the program, start by taking your seven-site skinfold body composition test. This will establish your baseline, or the benchmark against which you will compare all subsequent test results. Go to our website, enter your data, calculate your body composition, print out your result, and save it in a binder or file. Once you have established your baseline and have a basic understanding of the components of body composition, we recommend that you do the full seven-site skinfold body composition test once a .week. By saving your body composition printouts, you will document your progress. You will see trends that will help you understand how your body is responding to the behavioral changes you are making—and how to make effective adjustments to accelerate your progress. Taking your thigh and navel skinfold each morning will give you a "snapshot" of the direction in which you are headed. Your weekly seven-site readings will give you the full picture.

Tracking the changes in your body fat percentage, pounds of lean body mass, and pounds of fat will tell you what's really going on in your body. This will tell you which adjustments you need to make in your process (eating, exercise, water, sleep, etc.) in order to attain your ideal body weight.

Let's look at some of the possible outcomes of your weekly body composition tests and what they tell you.

With your initial body composition test, you should notice several things, beginning with your actual body fat percent. Next might be your ideal body weight. But a very important number is your lean body mass. How many pounds of fat-free weight do you have? And how does your actual lean body mass compare to this chart.

Minimum Lean Body Mass					
Women					
Height	5'0"	5'1"	5'2"	5'3"	5'4"	5'5"
Pounds	70-86	73-89	75-91	78-93	81-96	83-99
Height	5'6"	5'7"	5'8"	5'9"	5'10"	
Pounds	86-102	90-105	93-109	95-115	98-119	

Men						
Height	5'5"	5'6"	5'7"	5'8"	5'9"	
Pounds	108-120	110-125	112-129	118-132	122-137	
Height	5'10"	5'11"	6'0"	6'1"	6'2"	6'3"
Pounds	127-145	133-153	137-163	140-168	143-176	145-183

It is very common for women to be over-fat and under-muscled. This is a common outcome of dieting. If you discover that you are, in fact, under-muscled, then consistently getting forty to fifty grams of lean, complete protein with each of your meals becomes even more important. In fact, it is not unusual for under-muscled women to put on a fair amount of muscle relatively quickly. If they have been under-eating lean, complete protein and getting little or no exercise, their muscles will be very responsive. But not to worry. This initial surge of muscle will not continue. You are not going to become overly muscular. It is difficult for most men to put on much muscle, let alone women. But you will become stronger, more toned, and healthier. And your lean body mass *is* your metabolism, so putting on a little muscle is a positive thing.

Another issue may arise if you are already lean. How do you calculate your ideal body weight if you are leaner than 15 percent body fat for a man or 22 percent body fat for a woman right from the start? Simple. To calculate an ideal body fat percentage lower than 15 percent or 22 percent, take your goal body fat percentage and subtract that percentage from 100 percent. Then divide your actual lean body mass by that number. For example, let's say you are a two hundred–pound man with 12 percent body fat on your initial body composition test, but you would like to be 10 percent body fat. At two hundred pounds and 12 percent body fat, that means you have 176 pounds of lean body mass. Take your lean body mass (176 pounds) and divide that by the 90 percent (100 percent minus 10 percent). That number is .9, or 90 percent. 176 divided by .9 equals 195.56. Assuming you keep your lean body mass the same (176 pounds) and just lose body fat, your ideal body weight at 10 percent would be 195.56 pounds.

For a woman, let's say you were 20 percent body fat on your initial test, but you would like to be 15 percent body fat. And let's say you weigh 120 pounds. At 120 pounds and 20 percent body fat, you would have 96 pounds of lean mass. 100 percent minus 15 percent is .85, or 85 percent. 96 divided by .85 equals 112.94 pounds. Assuming you keep your lean body mass constant and just lose body fat, your ideal body weight at 15 percent would be 112.94 pounds.

To help you better understand what the changes in different components of your body composition results mean, let's go through the ten possible outcomes, one by one, and explain the possible causes of each outcome. The following ten outcomes are prioritized from most desirable (the best possible outcome) to the least desirable.

1. **Lose weight – Lose fat – Gain lean body mass (muscle):** To lose weight, lose body fat, and gain muscle simultaneously is the best possible and most desirable outcome. This is your straight-A report card. You are doing everything correctly and accurately. Getting leaner is a multi-factorial, ongoing learning process. You can't just do one thing. Getting leaner means you're doing an optimal combination of behaviors such as: staying consistently well hydrated; consistently eating a clean, balanced diet; exercising consistently; and consistently getting seven to nine hours of sound sleep. We deliberately used the word *consistently*. The ability to behave in a consistent manner over time is an important part of getting and staying lean. Your body does not lie. Consistency is an important component of success in life. Stability and consistency. If you are reasonably conscientious with our program, this is the result you will get most weeks. If you get sloppy with your program, your body and your skinfolds will reflect your behavior right away. Stay on track and your body will reward you with consistently positive feedback.

2. **Body weight stays the same – Lose fat – Gain lean body mass (muscle):** This outcome underscores the value of body composition testing. If you were only weighing yourself on your scale, you would think you have made no progress and might even feel a bit discouraged. But if you see this result, you should feel elated because, again, you are doing everything accurately and correctly. Any time you lose fat and simultaneously gain muscle, that is A work, and you deserve to feel proud. This is one aspect of getting leaner that sometimes surprises people: You do not necessarily have to lose any weight in order to get leaner. Take a moment and think this through. If you gain one pound

of muscle and you simultaneously lose one pound of fat, your weight on your scale has not changed at all. But you are definitely leaner. In fact, as you get leaner, you will notice that your weight loss will slow down, and at times will even stop all together, but you will continue to get leaner. Your clothes will continue to get looser. Your clothes don't lie. And you will see positive changes in your mirror. Your body will look more attractive.

3. **Gain weight – Lose fat – Gain lean body mass (muscle):** How can you gain weight and get leaner? Again, think it through. If you lose fat and gain muscle, but you gain *more* muscle than the fat you lost, your overall weight will go up. Again, your clothes will get looser. Why? A pound of muscle takes up less space than a pound of fat. This will not happen very often. It would be a good idea to cut back your carbohydrate calories just a little. Just enough so you lose about half a pound a week. Nothing drastic.

4. **Gain weight – Fat stays the same – Gain lean body mass (muscle):** If you gain weight, but the only weight you gain is muscle weight, that is a positive outcome. I remember a classic case of this very combination. We were underwater weighing at a chain of women's health clubs in the San Joaquin Valley here in California. At one particular club in Bakersfield, we always got a huge turnout and scheduled multiple test days. One of the female aerobics instructors had been tested three months earlier. In the intervening three months, she had worked hard to get as lean as she could. On the first day of testing, we retested her. Her initial results showed that she had lost weight, lost fat, but had also lost a lot of muscle so her body fat percent did not improve much. She had worked so hard that she was disappointed in her results, to the point of tears. As I explained her results and observed her emotional reaction, I asked her a few questions about her training, her eating, and how many classes she taught a week. It quickly became apparent to me that she was over-trained and under-carbed. Yes, this rarely but sometimes happens. She had actually cut her carbs too hard. I told her to go home, get a lot of rest, really carb up, and drink a lot of water. I told her to come back on the third and last day of our testing. Three days later, she had actually gained weight, but all of the weight she gained was muscle weight. As a result, her weight was up several pounds, but

her body fat had dropped dramatically. And she had gained back all the muscle she had apparently lost and more. What was going on? The first day I tested her, she was glycogen depleted. Glycogen is the stored form of glucose. Glycogen is stored in your muscles and in your liver. Glycogen is an integral part of your lean body mass (your muscles, bones, organs, and the fluids of your body). I could also tell from my experience of testing literally tens of thousands of clients that there was no way she was as fat as her initial retest said she was. I correctly guessed that she was over-trained and glycogen depleted. Needless to say, she was thrilled with her new, more accurate results. I tell this story to underscore what a blunt instrument a scale alone is and what misleading information your weight on a scale can be. Body composition testing gives you the only true and biologically accurate picture of what's really going on with your body. Again, this does not happen very often. For most people, it is a good idea to cut back your carbohydrate calories until you lose about half a pound a week.

5. **Gain weight – Gain fat – Gain lean body mass (muscle):** Your first impression may be that this is not a positive result. But the reason we put this particular result where we did is because this is the last of the combinations in which you gain muscle. Gaining muscle—that is, enhancing your lean body mass—is always a positive result. Your lean body mass is your metabolic engine. It is your lean body mass that burns calories and burns fat. It is also your lean body mass that gives your body strength and tone. Your lean body mass is gold. One of the hallmarks of aging is frailty. The last thing you want is to become frail. Being weak and frail severely circumscribes your life and the activities you can participate in. Your bones are an integral component of your lean body mass. You can have strong, healthy bones all your life. You never have to become that bent-over, old person. Poor posture is simply a sign of neglect. Use it or lose it. The time to start using and stimulating your body is now. You will feel better and look better now, and you will be making a huge investment in aging successfully. But again, any time you gain weight, your body is telling you that you are slightly overeating. Cut back your calories just enough so you only lose about half a pound a week. Keep your lean, complete protein intake high, your healthy fat at a moderate level, and your low glycemic load carbohydrates under control.

6. **Gain weight – Gain fat – Lean body mass (muscle) stays the same:** In this outcome, at least you do not lose lean body mass (muscle). But this outcome indicates you are both overeating and over-carbing. The key is to dial back your calories, *especially* your carbohydrate calories, until you are consistently losing about half a pound a week.

7. **Lose weight – Lose fat – Lose lean body mass (muscle):** In this outcome, you are under-eating both calories and protein. Slightly increase your calorie intake. All or most of your caloric increase should come from lean, complete protein.

8. **Weight stays the same – Gain fat – Lose lean mass (muscle):** This outcome may be caused by a couple of things. The fact that your weight stays the same indicates that you are eating the optimal number of calories. The fact that you gained fat but lost muscle tells you that you are over-eating carbs and under-eating lean, complete protein. A simple adjustment of your protein to carb ratio will correct this outcome and get you back on course. Keep your calories the same, but *increase* your intake of lean, complete protein and *decrease* your intake of slow-burning carbs.

9. **Lose weight – Gain fat – Lose lean mass (muscle):** Any time you lose weight, you are under-eating calories. That is what it takes to lose weight and fat. You should slightly under-eat calories. But if you are under-eating calories while over-eating carbs relative to your intake of lean, complete protein, you may lose weight while gaining fat and losing muscle. The answer: Adjust your protein to carb ratio. Keep your calorie intake constant, but *increase* your intake of lean, complete protein to protect your lean body mass and *decrease* your carbs. This will accelerate your fat loss.

10. **Gain weight – Gain fat – Lose lean body mass (muscle):** Any time you gain weight, you are eating more calories than your body needs. The solution here is to reduce your calorie intake slightly (no more than three hundred to five hundred calories per day or exercise a little more—or a combination of both that adds up to three hundred to five hundred calories per day), but *don't* cut your lean protein intake. Instead, reduce your carb intake (and perhaps your fat intake as well).

Food and Your Mood

Sugar is addictive. Sugar (carbohydrate) is depressing. If you feel depressed and/or anxious, chances are you are eating more carbohydrates than *your* body and *your* brain can tolerate. Sugar lowers your impulse threshold. This can manifest itself with an act as simple as buying a candy bar as you go through the checkout stand at the supermarket, or it can manifest itself as an outburst of anger and rage at someone in your family (your spouse and/or your children). Sugar gives us a hair trigger, and at the same time, sugar withdrawal can make us angry, irritable, and impatient. If you suffer from depression, anxiety, and/or episodes of rage, take a look at your sugar/carb intake.

My mother was addicted to sugar all her life. She was hysterical at times, angry, and lashed out with vicious, emotionally hurtful attacks on those around her. My mother gained weight all her life. She became diabetic and eventually died of cancer at fifty-seven. She never escaped the tyranny of sugar. My mother was depressed and profoundly unhappy the entire time I knew her. She was a chain smoker and huge coffee drinker. When she wasn't terrorizing our household, she was often in bed with the drapes drawn and the bedroom door closed. Sugar is great for instant gratification, but the long-term cost is huge. Sugar destroys your health and your relationships. It is impossible to build a joyful, meaningful life when you are addicted to sugar.

Blood Testing

One of the best ways to listen to your body is through regular blood testing. Your blood results are the net-net of your health. We recommend that you establish a baseline by getting a full and comprehensive set of blood panels as soon as you can. Please see the Resources section for a practical and accurate source. Then retest every six to twelve months until your blood values are optimal and stable. Like with your body composition (your body fat percentage), the goal is to gain conscious, deliberate control over your blood values. A comprehensive set of blood panels should include the following:

Lipid Panel
Total Cholesterol: 180-199 mg/dl
LDL: 0-99 mg/dl (lower is better)
HDL: > 55 mg/dl (higher is better)
Triglycerides: 0-99 mg/dl (lower is better)

Inflammation Markers:
CRP (C-Reactive Protein)
Men: < .55 mg/L (lower is better)
Women: < 1.5 mg/L (lower is better)

Fasting Insulin: 6-27 uIU/mL (lower is better)
Hemoglobin A1C: < 4.5% (lower is better)
Fibrinogen: 200-300 mg/dl

Hormones:
Thyroid:
TSH: .35-2.1 uIU/mL
T 3: 2.80-3.2 pg/mL
T 4: 4.5-12 ug/dl

DHEA-Sulfate:
Men: 400-500 ug/dl
Women: 150-350 ug/dl

Estradiol:
Men: 10-30 pg/ml
Women: 20-200 pg/ml

Progesterone:
Men: 3.8-5.2 ng/mL
Women: 4.4-28 ng/mL

Testosterone:
Men: Free: 25-35 pg/ml
Total: 241-827 ng/dL
Women: Free: 1.4-2.2 pg/mL
Total: 14-76 ng/dL

Pregnenolone:
Men: 20-180 ng/dL
Women: 20-200 ng/dl

Other Blood Factors:

PSA (Men Only): 0-2.6 ng/ml (less than 1.0 is optimal; lower is better)

IGF-1: 87-225 ng/mL

Fasting Glucose: 70-85 mg/dl

Homocysteine: < 7.2 umol/L (lower is better)

Vitamin D: 40-80 ng/mL

Optimal hormone levels seem to be a neglected area in our culture. As you age, your hormone levels decline. Declining hormone levels are a natural part of the aging process. The consequences of suboptimal hormone levels show up in the form of menopausal and andropausal symptoms. In the past, there was not much you could do about it, other than learn to live with a less than optimal quality life. But today, you have some positive options: bio-identical hormone replacement.

For women, progesterone cream is often a good place to start, provided your progesterone levels are less than optimal on your blood tests and you are suffering from menopausal symptoms. Pro Fem cream (2.5 percent progesterone, 5 mg per pump) applied twice a day will help with hot flashes, anxiety, and irritability. Since this is considered a supplement, you can purchase this without a prescription. Estrogen (Estradiol), on the other hand, is a bit trickier and will require a doctor's prescription. Although this seems to be the place most physicians start, we feel that many women (especially those who are overweight) are actually in a state of estrogen dominance. Estrogen dominance can contribute to many hormone-dependent cancers, so we advise you to take the absolute least amount you need to feel better, and proceed with caution. Discuss this with your physician.

Free testosterone, plus T3 and T4 to supplement your thyroid function, are two other hormone replacement medications that are quite often beneficial. These are important for both men and women. With a doctor's prescription, you can take small amounts of these hormones to replenish your less-than-optimal levels. Often, the synergy of these two will make a profound difference in the quality of your life.

The most effective form of thyroid supplement is Armour, which is a natural mix of both T3 and T4. It does not take much. Start low and slowly and incrementally increase your dose until your feel like "yourself" again.

Optimal levels of free testosterone are not only important for overall well-being, but optimal levels of testosterone are essential if you want to have a healthy, fully functioning brain and a strong, healthy heart. For women, the most effective way to optimize your free testosterone levels is with a cream you apply in the morning, as women usually only need a tiny amount compared to men, and usually only once a day. For men, the most effective way to optimize your free testosterone levels is with sublingual lozenges. Men usually need more and need to take three lozenges a day: first thing in the morning, late morning, and late afternoon. Although, there are many other options out there (gels, creams, injections, etc.), we have found that sublingual lozenges will give you the most even levels of free testosterone. Testosterone cannot be taken in a pill. Sublingual lozenges, however, dissolve either under the tongue or via the buccal mucosa, so they are assimilated directly through the capillaries.

Men (especially if they are overweight) may also find they are producing excess estrogen. This is most commonly seen in men whose total testosterone levels appear optimal, but their free testosterone is suboptimal. If this is the case, make sure you check your estradiol levels. This may mean your testosterone is aromatizing (converting) to estrogen. Check with your physician.

Again, start slow, and increase your dose incrementally until you feel like "yourself" again. For some men, this means they begin to smile, laugh, and enjoy life again. Women quite often report this feeling as well. Once you discover the optimal amount for you, the key is to take it consistently every day. As you get older, every five years or so, you may need to slightly increase the dose.

The lifestyle outlined in this book is designed to optimize your blood results. Establishing your baseline values, plus regular retesting, will clearly show you in black and white numbers if what you are doing is enough, or if you have to be more aggressive in your behavioral changes. It is that simple. All these blood values are in your control. You just have to be mature enough to make the behavioral changes to get you there. It is not easy. But that is why real health has value. Anything of value has a price. The higher the value, the higher the price. There is no free lunch.

Chapter 19

Manage YOUR Setbacks

Tis folly to cry for spilt milk.
                                        —Jonathan Swift, 1738

Once you set your outcome goal, commit to your plan, and create your home base, your next step is to begin testing your process. As you begin to live your process, setbacks will show up. Setbacks are alarms or signals alerting you to a flaw in your process.

Jonathan Swift is one of my favorite writers. As part of an essay he wrote on clichés in 1738, Swift satirized people's use of language. He used the expression, "Tis folly to cry for spilt milk," so the concept of crying over spilt milk must to have been around long enough that it was already a cliché in 1738. This expression is not new, but its meaning still escapes some people today. The concept is: Once an event is in the past, there is literally nothing you can do to change it, so get over it. Move on. Stop living your life by looking in the rearview mirror all the time. Feeling guilty or bad about yourself over something in the past is a waste of time and energy. What's done is done.

To err is human, as the saying goes. You are going to make mistakes. You are going to get off track. How you handle your mistakes makes all the difference. One of the most important and useful questions you should continually ask yourself is, "What is the reality of the situation?" Once you have made a mistake and eaten something unhealthy, the reality is simple: It's in the past and cannot be changed.

You only have so much psychic energy. Don't waste your limited psychic energy beating yourself up over something you cannot change. Instead, take a deep breath. Regain your composure. Regain your perspective. What can you do *now*? First, don't compound your error. Just because you have made one mistake, don't use it as an excuse to blow your entire day or night. Nip your self-destructive behavior in the bud. Notice your circumstances. How did you get yourself into this fix? What is the lesson or lessons to be learned? Was it the location? Was it a particular room in your house? Was it a particular food? Was it a particular combination of food and location? Are you and your partner on the same page? Was it your mood? Were you overly hungry? Were you overly tired? Were you feeling lonely? Were you feeling depressed? Were you emotionally hurt? Were you angry? Did you have a fight?

One key to handling your setbacks is to avoid wild swings of behavior. Avoid reacting or over-reacting. Instead, respond to your setback thoughtfully, calmly, and deliberately. Regain rational control. The Joe Dillon Difference is a rational, reality-based lifestyle.

Your home is one place where you do have some control. Learn from your setbacks and change those things you can change. For example, you may find that you can't stop eating a certain food, even though it may be healthy, such as raw nuts. Maybe you are okay with almonds, but can't stop eating raw walnuts or raw pecans, or vice versa. Intellectually, it might not make any sense. But the tangible results don't lie. The safest approach is to eliminate the food or foods you can't stop eating, no matter how healthy they are.

Maybe it is a situation that set you off. For example, maybe you tend to overeat when you watch television and have easy access to an open container of food like a bowl of cherries or a bowl of raw almonds. Maybe you find that when you get home late and you're tired, you end up mindlessly overeating while watching sports highlights. Distracted eating can be a big problem for some people. Have only a limited amount of food when you are watching television. Get your home as close to bulletproof as you can. To prevent setbacks, stay aware of your triggers and your trigger foods, and then eliminate them. Keep refining your process.

Once you have created a strong, healthy environment and routine at home, you have taken the first step. A clean house is crucial to your success. Then you are ready to expand your horizons. Your car is your home away from home. Is your car clean and stocked with your healthy items? Be proactive. Think through each situation the best you can. Then refine your process when a setback shows up. You get caught in rush hour traffic and you're starving. Be better prepared next time. A very effective way of dealing with setbacks is to create checklists. Create a simple checklist on your computer. Then as setbacks show up, refine your checklist to prevent future setbacks.

Your work environment will pose a whole new set of potential setbacks you never thought of. Dealing with lunches, either with the people you work with or business lunches with clients, can be tricky. Business travel ups the ante even more. You have to deal with challenges such as airports, airplanes, being bored and tired during layovers, rental cars, hotel rooms, room service menus, eating out at restaurants on the road, and being lonely in your room. Having learned the hard way, I almost always stay at a hotel with a kitchen in the room, including at least a microwave and a refrigerator. That way I can pick up the food and water I need at a grocery store and eat pretty clean even on the road. I continue to refine my business travel checklist.

Sometimes the toughest situations are the ones we least expect. Going to a friend's home or a family gathering can be a major challenge. Over the years, our family has built up all kinds of unconscious expectations about our behavior, including what we eat. They may not know or understand that you are making a change. They may be confused when you don't eat three helpings of your aunt's key lime pie like you usually do. Families can exert tremendous pressure and trigger a setback. Friends may try to be helpful and prepare foods they think are healthy when, in fact, they are not healthy at all. They just don't have the kind of information that you have now.

You will always encounter situations you did not foresee. The challenge at these moments is to be resourceful. Look around you. Assess the reality of the situation. What are the viable alternatives? The probability is that none of your alternatives will be perfect. Your job at that point is to choose the best of the real alternatives available to you at the time. Sometimes the choice is choosing the least of the worst. Be honest with yourself and choose the alternative that is most consistent with the lifestyle you espouse to. Improvise. Use your imagination. Maybe they served you chicken, but it's covered in sauce. Maybe the "healthy" salad they made especially for you is drenched in a thick, creamy dressing. Sometimes you just have to surrender and count this meal as one of your treat meals. This is all part of your learning process. Do the best you can in the given circumstances, but then think through how you might have prevented getting into this situation in the first place. Could you have called ahead and explained your new diet? Sometimes you can offer to bring a dish that you know is healthy, so you will have at least something to eat without hurting anyone's feelings. What will you do next time to avoid this problem in the future? As you work at it, you will build a repertoire of tools and behaviors that will keep you on track, or close to it, most of the time. Avoid making the same mistake twice.

Setbacks illuminate the vulnerable points in your process. This is the learning process. Rather than being discouraging, setbacks provide invaluable information. After each setback, retreat to the safety and security of your home base, and shore up your process. Think through your process again and figure out how to prevent the setback you just experienced. Then, when you venture out again, see if your new, updated process works better than your last one. If you are persistent, over time you will develop a nearly bulletproof process. You will be ready for any eventuality, and the only breaks in your process will be the ones you consciously decide to take, such as your treat meals. This is the way you gain control over your behavior and your body—and how you build confidence in yourself.

Love is perfect kindness. Part of getting lean is to love yourself properly. Nurturing yourself is how you get lean. Being harsh on yourself is a short-term, quick-fix approach to your problem. In business management, there are two theories on how to manage people: Theory X and Theory Y. Theory X is the iron-fisted, punitive approach to managing people. Driving people hard, with no compassion, will get better results in the short run, but ultimately this method fails. Why? Because people will only work hard when the tough boss is around. Theory X does not instill self-responsibility and pride. Theory Y is about positive reinforcement. It's about rewarding constructive behavior. Give praise and recognition to those who are doing their jobs well. It takes longer for Theory Y to produce results, but it is far more effective in the long run. Why? Because positive reinforcement works. People thrive on recognition, and people who feel good about themselves are more constructive. Punitive behavior just leads to resentment and poor self-esteem. Learn how to be a good manager of yourself.

Look for your own positive, constructive behavior and reward yourself. Nonfood rewards are best. Be kind to yourself, and the wild swings in your behavior and your weight will disappear.

Loving maturity and emotional stability are the answer. Consistent, constructive behavior is the answer. But you also have to recognize your dark side. You have a self-destructive, neurotic side. *Your* body does not lie. Your neurotic (self-destructive) side is not going to go away. The key is to recognize and acknowledge your self-destructive side and to circumscribe it. That is the main reason you need to keep your house clean. Don't tempt fate. Keep a tight rein on your self-destructive side. Avoid people who feed your self-destructive side. Avoid places that feed your self-destructive side. Don't set yourself up for a fall. For example, instead of hanging out at a bar, go to the gym. Bars are not constructive places, and bars are not filled with constructive people. Most people at bars are lonely, depressed people. Gyms are constructive places, filled with people doing constructive things. People in gyms are building something. People in gyms are building their strength, their health, and their endurance. People in gyms have positive goals and are self-disciplined. Positive, goal-oriented people are the kind of people you want in your life. Optimistic, goal-oriented people will help you accomplish your goals by their example, their discipline, and their energy.

You are never going to get the body you want in a bar, whereas a gym is an environment conducive to health and fitness. A gym has positive energy. At a gym, you can see people who have what you want: a lean, healthy body. At a gym, you can find role models. At a gym you can find people who inspire you. At a gym, you can see people your own age who are in great shape. At a gym, you can see concrete examples of what is possible.

There is a line from a Bob Dylan song that says something about the fact that there is no success like failure and that failure is no success at all. I think what he means is that you will often learn more from your mistakes than from your successes. Sometimes you need to learn the hard way, meaning that sometimes you need a wake-up call. You just hope that the wake-up call is not so severe that the damage is long-lasting. If you pay attention, you will notice life giving you subtle, gentle messages about what you need to change. If at first you don't get it, life will up the ante. If you are in serious denial, sometimes life takes a proverbial two-by-four to your forehead. My father was a classic example. He got a million messages from all directions to stop smoking and take better care of himself. But my father was stubborn. So finally life gave him a wake-up call from which he never recovered: a massive heart attack that killed him at age forty-six. I was twenty years old. My father's death was a wake-up call for me, but I didn't get it at the time. I just felt devastated about how unfair life was. I didn't get the message until over ten years later, when I finally got my nutritional act together. And I am still not perfect. I still regress and behave in self-destructive ways. It is an ongoing battle.

When you experience a setback, this is the time to be your own best friend, to be your best coach, to re-parent yourself. It's okay if you are temporarily upset. But then say, "Oh well," and step back. Look for a pattern to see if there is something you are doing that is habitually putting you in a weak position. Try to discover the lesson or lessons. With renewed resolve, get right back on track and move forward. One of the great things about The Joe Dillon Difference is you have a clear track on which to run. When you get off track, get right back on as soon as you can. Life is full of curve balls. What separates successful people from unsuccessful people is that successful people bounce back from setbacks. Successful people get knocked down, but they get right back up. It's not how many times you get knocked down that counts. What counts is how many times you get back up. If you are an optimistic, goal-oriented person, you view setbacks as the exception, not the rule.

The Joe Dillon Difference is about self-responsibility. If you are going to get lean, it is going to be your fault. If you are not as lean now as you would like to be, it is waste of time to try to place the blame somewhere else. The Joe Dillon Difference lifestyle is between you and the person you see in the mirror. The Joe Dillon Difference is about who you are when no one is looking. The Joe Dillon Difference is between you and you. If you have a setback, you are ultimately responsible. The good news is that if you are responsible, you can do something about it. You are *not* a victim. It is *your* life and *you* are in control.

Chapter 20

Conclusion

It is because human metabolism is so sensitive to environmental cues that manipulative economic forces are now generating the current obesity epidemic.
—Jonathan C. K. Wells, PhD, *The Evolutionary Biology of Human Body Fatness: Thrift and Control, 2010*

You have just one life. You only have a finite amount of time. The past is gone forever. The future is promised to no one. What are *you* going to do with *your* time? Are you going to be a good steward of the gift of life you have been given? That is what we advocate, that you take the very best care of what you have been given, so you can enjoy the highest quality of life for as long as possible.

Unfortunately, you live at a time and in an environment that makes optimizing your health a major challenge. I am a twice-wounded combat marine who spent twelve and a half months in the jungle in South Vietnam. In combat, you learn very quickly to be hyper-vigilant all the time, or you don't survive. The realization that you are in a hostile environment is inescapable. Living in our modern obesogenic environment is similar to jungle combat. You must learn to protect yourself at all times. You must learn there are very few people to whom you can trust your health and life. You must learn that most people are incompetent about their life and health. If you have any doubts, look at their bodies. The body never lies.

You must learn there are very few safe places. Hopefully, you learn all this before you get killed. Many marines in South Vietnam died within their first thirty days in-country. They did not learn fast enough how to keep themselves alive. Combat is the ultimate Darwinian world. You either adapt or you die. In civilian life, it is the same, just not as dramatic. If you don't learn, you are victimized by your environment; you get fat and sick; and you die prematurely.

So first and foremost, this book is a head's-up, a wake-up call. We are sounding the alarm for you to keep your head down and watch out for land mines and booby-traps. This book is a reminder that the Black Box of Conventional Wisdom (marketing) is someone else's agenda for someone else's benefit. The Black Box is *not* for your benefit. In fact, the Black Box is the opposite. The Black Box is intent on exploiting you. The Black Box does its best to manipulate you. If you don't know where you are going, any road will do. If you do not have your own clear agenda, you are living someone else's agenda.

There is no controversy about biological health and how to build optimal health. The 24/7 media circus is a superficial distraction. The fundamentals of optimal health are clear and settled. Evolutionary and molecular biology provide consensus scientific proof. And your own body confirms those facts. Simply and consistently provide your body with the biological essentials (oxygen; water; lean, complete protein; healthy, raw fat; low glycemic load carbohydrates; full-body aerobic exercise; optimal sleep; and some basic supplements) and your own body will give you all the proof you need. To document your results, follow our comprehensive program: Do a comprehensive set of blood panels every six to twelve months; weigh yourself, measure your waist and your navel and your thigh skinfolds every morning, and write down your results; and do your seven-site skinfold body composition test once a week to verify that you are losing fat and gaining muscle. It is that simple.

Why is it so hard? It is challenging to take good care of yourself because you are subjected to enormous pressures from corporate advertising; from government institutions such as the United States Department of Agriculture; and from your family, friends, and people you work with. These are all organizations that create the Black Box and/or people who are trapped in the Black Box. The most difficult people to resist are those who have no idea they are trapped in the Black Box. They are so full of conviction, and they apparently have no doubts. They seem so sure of themselves that you begin to question yourself. Don't. Instead, look at their bodies. Listen to *your* body. Your body is your touchstone.

To be lean and healthy in our obesogenic culture and environment, you have to be willing to go against the grain, to swim against the tide, to live outside the herd. Learn to think for yourself. Learn to be true to yourself. Do you want to live your life as an original, authentic life, or do you want to live a cookie-cutter life, someone else's idea of what your life should be?

The good life is what is good for *you*. The good life is not what is good for beer, pizza, or car sales. When you are being sold on the so-called good life, the question to ask yourself is: How does this benefit me in the long run? Learn to look beyond the immediate superficial circumstances and instead focus on *your* long-term goals. This is *your* life we are talking about here. Ask yourself: Do you really think the advertising people who created that beer ad on TV have the slightest idea who you are or care one bit about you and your life? Get real. They are professional manipulators trying to persuade you to spend your hard-earned money on a product to generate corporate profits.

There are a few clearly defined and simple steps in the process of losing weight. First and foremost, you must set a goal. Without a goal, you are just wandering aimlessly. Your first goal should be to attain 15 percent or 22 percent body fat (for men and women, respectively), if you are not there already. Do your seven-site skinfold body composition test, enter your data on our website, and print out your results. This will give you an ideal body weight based on your individual lean body mass. Your ideal body weight is your number one goal. Your ideal body weight will be recalculated each week you retest, based on changes in your lean body mass.

With this book, you have a clearly defined and an effective action plan to get you to your ideal body weight. Get your house clean. Create an environment that is conducive to your goals. Stock your house with water, and be prepared to stay well hydrated every day. Stock your house with lean, complete protein such as turkey, chicken, fish, egg whites, and whey protein isolate powder for your shakes. Make sure you have a dependable blender. Stock your house with low glycemic load carbohydrates such as leafy green and other vegetables, plus whole, fresh fruit. Stock your house with healthy fat, including molecularly distilled fish oil capsules and raw nuts. Based on consensus science, the ancestral diet consists of the following percentages based on percent of total calories:

- **50–60 percent lean, complete protein**

- **20–25 percent slow-burning carbohydrates**

- **20–25 percent raw, healthy fats**

These percentages translate into a simple meal template: a *fist* of lean, complete protein, combined with a *fist* of low glycemic load carbohydrates, combined with a *thumb* of raw fat. Follow this format for each of your four to six meals per day and limit your treat meals from one to no more than three per week, and you will make steady progress.

Schedule in thirty to forty-five minutes, three to five times a week, for your walks with light hand-weights. Stock your house with the basic supplements. Set up your schedule so you get an optimal amount of sleep each night. Work your process. Notice where your process breaks down (setbacks) and fine-tune your process accordingly. Be prepared for the long haul. Your first goal is to achieve your ideal weight. One of your long-term goals is to sustain your ideal weight for the rest of your long and healthy life.

The Black Box of Conventional Wisdom is all-encompassing. It takes a lot of energy to escape the gravitational pull of the Black Box. Most people don't even realize they are trapped in the Black Box. Of those who do wake up enough to realize they are trapped, most of them never escape. Working to avoid being sucked back into the vortex of the Black Box is like paddling your canoe upstream all the time. The current never gets tired, and the current never quits. Complacency is your constant opponent. Drop your guard, and you will get swept down the stream into the whirlpool of the Black Box.

Symptoms of the Black Box are everywhere. Here are a few examples: There are literally hundreds of television channels but nothing worth watching; social networks have never been bigger, and yet people are more lonely and isolated than ever; most people are overfed but undernourished; and since the invention of agriculture, human beings have gotten smaller and sicker and our brains are over 10 percent smaller than the brains of pre-agricultural humans.

Ultimately, listen to *your* body. Trust *your* direct experience: your scale, your tape measure, your skinfolds, your energy levels, and your mental acuity. Stay firmly rooted in the biological reality of your body and you won't go wrong. Once you escape the Black Box and its silliness, it will be clear what's really important. It is like when the first Apollo mission left the gravitational pull of the earth and the astronauts could look back and see the entire earth for the very first time: a beautiful blue and green orb in the vast blackness of space. Seeing our earth from that perspective for the first time made all the bickering back on earth over borders, etc., seem petty. Seeing the earth from that perspective makes you realize we are all literally in the same boat. Once you escape the gravitational pull of the Black Box, you will see how important *your* life is and how important it is to take the very best care of your life that you can. Your new lifestyle is real and will give you the body, the energy, the health, and the enthusiasm you are looking for. It is up to you. We know you can do it.

Resources

Appendix A

Optimal Sources of Water

■ Distilled Water

■ Filtered Water

■ Spring Water

■ Sparkling Water

■ Herbal Teas (made with one of the above waters)

■ Decaf Coffee (made with one of the above waters)

■ Decaf Tea (made with one of the above waters)

Optimal Sources of Lean, Complete Protein

- 100% Whey Protein Isolate Powder
- Egg Whites
- Wild Game (venison, buffalo, elk, moose, etc.)
- Salmon, Ahi Tuna
- Turkey (white meat, dark meat, no skin)
- Fish (all kinds)
- Tuna (water-packed only)
- Chicken (white meat only, no skin)
- Shellfish (oysters, mussels, clams, lobster, shrimp, crab)
- Nonfat Dairy (nonfat milk, nonfat cheese, nonfat cottage cheese, nonfat plain yogurt)

Low Glycemic Load Carbohydrates: Choose One

- Leafy Green Vegetables (unlimited)

- Vegetables (1-2 cups per meal, fresh or frozen, NOT canned)

- Fruit (1/2 to 1 cup per meal, fresh or frozen, unsweetened)

- Yams, Sweet Potatoes (1/2 to 1 cup cooked per meal)

- Beans, Peas, Lentils (1/2 cup cooked per meal)

- Whole Grains (1/2 cup cooked per meal)

    Wild Rice
    Brown Rice (short grain or long grain)
    Corn
    Wheat
    Rye
    Barley
    Oat Groats

Raw, Healthy Fats and Oils:
A Thumb or a Tablespoon

- Molecularly Distilled Fish Oil (6-12 capsules per day)

- Raw Seeds: Flax, Sunflower, Sesame, Pumpkin

- Raw Seed Oil: Raw, Organic Flax Seed Oil
  Note: Must be refrigerated

- Raw Tree Nuts: Almonds, Cashews, Walnuts, Pecans, Hazelnuts
  Note: Peanuts are NOT nuts—peanut butter is junk food

- Raw Nut Butter: Raw Almond Butter, Raw Cashew Butter
  Note: must be refrigerated

- Avocado (1 slice—about an eighth)

- Olive Oil: Extra virgin is the highest quality

Name:

Goal:

TheJoeDillonDifference.com

Daily Measurements Log

Today's Date	Weight in Pounds	Waist Inches	Navel Skinfold	Thigh Skinfold

TheJoeDillonDifference.com

Daily Food, Water and Exercise Log

Name:

Goal:

Today's Date	Breakfast	Mid-Morning	Lunch	Mid-Afternoon	Dinner	Pre-Sleep	Water	Workout

Appendix B

Recommended Reading

Anderson, Bob. *Stretching: For Everyday Fitness and for Running, Tennis, Racquetball, Cycling, Swimming, Golf, and Other Sports.* Shelter Publications, Inc., Bolinas, California, 1980.

Barker, David. *Nutrition in the Womb: How Better Nutrition During Development Will Prevent Heart Disease, Diabetes and Stroke.* The Developmental Origins of Health and Disease, 2008.

Bass, Clarence. *Ripped: The Sensible Way to Achieve Ultimate Muscularity.* Ripped Enterprises, 1980.

Brown, Janet. *Charles Darwin: Voyaging.* Princeton University Press, 1995.

Brown, Janet. *Charles Darwin: The Power of Place.* Princeton University Press, 2002.

Burke, Edmund R. *Optimal Muscle Performance and Recovery.* Avery, New York, 2003.

Csikszentmihalyi, Mihayli, *Flow: The Psychology of Optimal Experience.* Harper Perennial, 1990.

Darwin, Charles. *The Voyage of the Beagle: Charles Darwin's Journal of Research.* Pacific Publishing Studio, 1839.

Darwin, Charles. *The Origin of Species*. Sterling, New York, 1859.

Darwin, Charles. *The Descent of Man*. A Plume Book, 1871.

DeGrasse Tyson PhD, Neil. *Origins: Fourteen Billion Years of Cosmic Evolution*. NOVA, WBGH, Boston, 4 hour DVD, 2004.

Desalle, Rob, and Ian Tattersall. *Human Origins: What Bones and Genomes Tell Us About Ourselves*. Texas A & M University Press, College Station, Texas, 2008.

Diamond, Jared. *The Third Chimpanzee: The Evolution and Future of the Human Animal*. Harper Perennial, 1992.

Edelson, Edward. *Gregor Mendel: And the Roots of Genetics*. Oxford University Press, 1999.

Erasmus, Udo. *Fats That Heal, Fats That Kill*. Alive Books, 1993.

Finch, Caleb E. *The Biology of Human Longevity: Inflammation, Nutrition, and Aging in the Evolution of Lifespans*. Academic Press, 2007.

Food, Nutrition, Physical Activity, and the Prevention of Cancer: a Global Perspective. A Project of the World Cancer Research Fund International, 517 pages, 2007.

Gibbons, Ann. *The First Human: The Race to Discover Our Earliest Ancestors*. Anchor Books, New York, 2006.

Gluckman, Peter, and Mark Hanson. *The Fetal Matrix: Evolution, Development and Disease*. Cambridge University Press, 2005.

Gluckman, Peter, and Mark Hanson. *Mismatch: The Lifestyle Diseases Timebomb*. Oxford University Press, 2008.

Gluckman, Peter, Alan Beedle, and Mark Hanson. *Principles of Evolutionary Medicine*. Oxford University Press, 2009.

Hager, Thomas. *Force of Nature: The Life of Linus Pauling*. Simon & Schuster, New York, 1995.

Halberstam, David. *The Amateurs: The Story of Four Young Men and*

Their Quest for an Olympic Gold Medal. Fawcell Books, New York, 1985.

Hall, Sara. *Drawn to the Rhythm: A Passionate Life Reclaimed.* W. W. Norton and Company, New York, 2002.

Hawks PhD, John. *The Rise of Humans: Great Scientific Debates.* The Teaching Company, 12 hour DVD course, 2011.

Hudson, Fredric M. *The Adult Years: Mastering the Art of Self-Renewal.* Jossey-Bass Publishers, San Francisco, 1991.

Jablonka, Eva, and Marion J. Lamb. *Evolution in Four Dimensions: Genetic, Epigenetic, Behavioral, and Symbolic Variation in the History of Life.* Massachusetts Institute of Technology, Cambridge, Massachusetts, 2005.

Johanson, Donald C., and Maitland Edey. *Lucy: The Beginnings of Humankind.* Simon & Schuster, 1981.

Johanson, Donald, and James Shreeve. *Lucy's Child: The Discovery of a Human Ancestor.* William Morrow and Company, Inc., New York, 1989.

Johanson, Donald, and Blake Edgar. *From Lucy to Language.* Simon & Schuster, New York, 2006.

Johanson, Donald C., and Kate Wong. *Lucy's Legacy: The Quest for Human Origins.* Three Rivers Press, New York, 2009.

Kandel, Eric R. *In Search of Memory: The Emergence of a New Science of Mind.* W. W. Norton and Company, New York, 2006.

Kiesling, Stephen. *The Shell Game: Reflections on Rowing and the Pursuit of Excellence.* Nordic Knight Press, Ashland, Oregon, 1982.

Klein, Richard G., and Blake Edgar. *The Dawn of Human Culture: A Bold New Theory of What Sparked the "Big Bang" of Human Consciousness.* John Wiley and Sons, Inc., 2002.

Klein, Richard G. *The Human Career: Human Biological and Cultural Origins.* The University of Chicago Press, Chicago, 2009.

Lambert, Craig. *Mind Over Water: Lessons on Life from the Art of Rowing.* Houghton Mifflin Company, Boston, 1998.

Larson, Joan Matthews. *Seven Weeks to Sobriety: The Proven Program to Fight Alcoholism Through Nutrition.* Ballantine Wellspring, New York, 1997.

Leakey, Richard, and Roger Lewin. *Origins Reconsidered: In Search of What Makes Us Human.* Random House, New York, 1992.

Levinson, Daniel J. *The Seasons of a Man's Life.* Alfred A. Knopf, New York, 1978.

Lindeberg, Staffan. *Food and Western Disease: Health and Nutrition from an Evolutionary Perspective.* Wiley-Blackwell, 2010.

Maas, James B. *Power Sleep: The Revolutionary Program That Prepares Your Mind for Peak Performance.* Harper Collins, 1998.

McKibben, Bill. *Long Distance: A Year of Living Strenuously.* Simon & Schuster, New York, 2000.

Medina, John. *Brain Rules: 12 Principles for Surviving and Thriving at Work, Home, and School.* Pear Press, 2008.

Miller, Philip Lee. *The Life Extension Revolution: The New Science of Growing Older Without Aging.* Bantam Books, 2006.

Neeson, Liam, narrator, *Evolution: Darwin's Dangerous Idea.* WGBH PBS, 2 hour DVD, 2001.

Northrup, Christiane. *The Wisdom of Menopause: Creating Physical and Emotional Health and Healing During the Change.* Bantam Books, New York, 2001.

Nova: *Cracking the Code of Life.* WGBH, Boston, 1 hour DVD, 2004.

Nova: *Becoming Human: How Early Hominids Lived and Evolved.* WGBH, Boston, 4 hour DVD, 2009.

Nowicki PhD, Stephen. *Biology: The Science of Life.* The Teaching Company, 36 hour DVD course, 2004.

Palmer, Douglas. *Origins: Human Evolution Revealed*. Mitchell Beazley, 2010.

Potts, Richard, and Christopher Sloan. *What Does It Mean To Be Human?* National Geographic Society, 2010.

Power, Michael L., and Jay Schulkin. *The Evolution of Obesity*. The Johns Hopkins University Press, Baltimore, 2009.

Sapolsky, Robert M. *Why Zebras Don't Get Ulcers: An Updated Guide to Stress, Stress-Related Disease, and Coping*. W. H. Freeman and Company, New York, 1998.

Sapolsky, Robert M. *A Primate's Memoir: A Neuroscientist's Unconventional Life Among the Baboons*. Scribner, New York, 2001.

Schwartz, Leonard. *Heavyhands: The Ultimate Exercise*. Little, Brown and Company, Boston, 1982.

Schwartz, Leonard. *The Heavyhands Walking Book: An Open Invitation to Convert Walking into a Lifelong Total Fitness Strategy*. Panaerobics Press, 1990.

Sheehan, George. *Running & Being: The Total Experience*. Warner Books, 1978.

Stringer, Chris, and Peter Andrews. *The Complete World of Human Evolution*. Thames & Hudson, London, 2005.

Tattersall, Ian. *Becoming Human: Evolution and Human Uniqueness*. Harcourt Brace and Company, New York, 1998.

Wells, Jonathan C. K. *The Evolutionary Biology of Human Body Fatness: Thrift and Control*. Cambridge University Press, 2010.

Wells, Spencer. *The Journey of Man: A Genetic Odyssey*. Random House, New York, 2002.

Wells PhD, Spencer. *Journey of Man: The Story of the Human Species*. PBS Home Video, 2 hour DVD, 2003.

Wilmore, Jack H., and David L. Costill. *Physiology of Sport and Exercise*. Human Kinetics, 1999.

Wrangham, Richard. *Catching Fire: How Cooking Makes Us Human*. Basic Books, New York, 2009.

Wright, Robert. *The Moral Animal: Why We Are the Way We Are: The New Science of Evolutionary Psychology*. Random House, New York, 1994.

Wright, Robert. *Nonzero: The Logic of Human Destiny*. Random House, New York, 2000.

Zimmer, Carl. *Evolution: The Triumph of an Idea*. Harper Perennial, 2002.

Zimmer, Carl. *Soul Made Flesh: The Discovery of the Brain—and How it Changed the World*. Free Press, New York, 2004.

Zimmer, Carl. *Smithsonian Intimate Guide to Human Origins*. Smithsonian Books, 2005.

Zimmer, Carl. *The Tangled Bank: An Introduction to Evolution*. Roberts and Company, Greenwood Village, Colorado, 2010.

Appendix C

Recommended Websites

Joe & Sandy's Website: TheJoeDillonDifference.com

Unlimited Free Seven-Site Skinfold Body Composition Testing

What you will learn:

Ideal Body Weight: What you should weigh based on your lean body mass.

Body Fat Percentage: How lean are you?

Lean Body Mass: Do you have enough muscle?

Order: Blood Testing: Comprehensive Blood Panels

Direct link to state-of-the-art blood testing.

Scheduled at a lab within minutes of your home or office.

Your blood results sent directly to you.

Order truly comprehensive blood panels at very reasonable prices now.

Order: Protein Powder

Now you understand the crucial importance of lean, complete protein.

Order the highest quality whey protein on the market.

The only totally 100% natural whey protein isolate powder on the market.

Order: Book

Share this rational, scientific, effective way of life with family, friends, and co-workers.

Join Now: Membership: one year or lifetime: Benefits to YOU:

- Major discounts on all of Joe and Sandy's products and services.
- Up to 24 Coaching Videos included FREE as part of your membership.
- Up to 24 MP3 Coaching downloads included FREE as part of your membership.
- Unlimited Downloads of useful tools included FREE as part of your membership.

staffanlindeberg.com

Paleolithic Diet in Medical Nutrition

Incorporating evolutionary biology in nutritional science. Staffan Lindeberg, MD, PhD, Department of Medicine, University of Lund, Sweden.

What is it?

Lean meat, fish, fruits, vegetables, root vegetables, eggs, nuts, etc.

What is it not?

Grains, dairy products, refined sugar, fats and oils. Today, these provide about 70 percent of the caloric intake in Western societies. And salt intake is much higher now.

Why bother?

It prevents heart disease, stroke and some forms of cancers and has a beneficial effect on overweight, digestive problems and more.

http://iho.asu.edu/

Institute of Human Origins

Becoming Human: 30 Years of Research and Discovery

The Institute of Human Origins brings together a diverse group of scientists in the investigation of human evolution and its contemporary relevance. Through innovative research, education, the sponsorship of scholarly interaction, the Institute fosters a multidisciplinary approach to the most important issues of the human trajectory.

> *"There is a desire amongst people to know about origins of all sorts of things … most importantly, origins of themselves."*
>
> —Don Johanson, PhD

eva.mpg.de

The Max Planck Institute for Evolutionary Anthropology

The Max Planck Institute for Evolutionary Anthropology unites scientists with various backgrounds (natural sciences and humanities) whose aim is to investigate the history of humankind from an interdisciplinary perspective with the help of comparative analyses of genes, cultures, cognitive abilities, languages, and social systems of past and present human populations, as well as those of primates closely related to human beings.

Department of Human Evolution

Led by Jean-Jacques Hublin, the Department of Human Evolution was founded in 2004 as part of the Max Planck Institute for Evolutionary Anthropology (MPI-EVA). The department primarily studies fossil hominins and aims to reconstruct their biology, behavior, and cultural evolution. Hominins are an extremely successful group of species that have expanded across the entire planet and have succeeded in coping in virtually all eco-geographical niches. Hominins have modified their environment to a spectacular extent, provoked one of the largest mass extinctions in the earth's history, and have developed some degree of control over their own genome and those of other species. For the first three or four million years of their evolution, like other mammals, hominins competed with other species and adapted to environmental changes primarily through biological adaptations; that is, by modifying their size, diet, locomotion and reproductive pattern. However, during the last two million years, the development of complex behavior related to the emergence of technology and, more broadly, to human culture has opened an entirely new chapter of primate evolution. Human evolution is unparalleled in life history because it is a bio-cultural process. What makes this process unique is the increasing importance of culture in the adaptive strategy of the species and, even more so, the increased interaction between culture and biology.

thesciencenetwork.org

The Science Network

Watch video interviews with the world's leading scientists talking about their cutting-edge research, including: evolution, aging, genetics, sleep, neuroscience, stem cells, and learning. Many of the authors of the recommended books and the research papers in the bibliography are interviewed on the Science Network talking about their current research.

bruceames.org

Bruce Ames, PhD

Cutting edge research on aging

Dr. Ames is a professor of biochemistry and molecular biology, University of California, Berkeley, and a senior scientist at Children's Hospital Oakland Research Institute (CHORI).

He is a member of the National Academy of Sciences and he served on its Commission on Life Sciences. He was a member of the board of directors of the National Cancer Institute, the National Cancer Advisory Board, from 1976 to 1982. He was the recipient of the General Motors Cancer Research Foundation Prize (1983), the Tyler Environmental Prize (1985), the Gold Medal Award of the American Institute of Chemists (1991), the Glenn Foundation Award of the Gerontological Society of America (1992), the Lovelace Institutes Award for Excellence in Environmental Health Research (1995), the Honda Prize of the Honda Foundation, Japan (1996), the Japan Prize, (1997), the Kehoe Award, American College of Occup. and Environ. Med. (1997), the Medal of the City of Paris (1998), the U.S. National Medal of Science (1998), The Linus Pauling Institute Prize for Health Research (2001), and the American Society for Microbiology Lifetime Achievement Award (2001).

His over 450 publications have resulted in his being among one of the most cited scientists in the world.

amnh.org/exhibitions/darwin/

American Museum of Natural History: Charles Darwin

Happiest at home with his notebooks and his microscope, he shunned the public eye. Controversy made him ill. The brilliant observer of nature kept his most original and revolutionary idea under wraps for decades. Yet, today, two centuries after Charles Darwin's birth, nearly everyone knows his name. What did Darwin do, and why does he matter so much?

Keenly observing nature in all its forms—from fossil sloths to mockingbirds, primroses to children—Darwin saw that we are all related. Every living thing shares an ancestry, he concluded, and the vast diversity of life on earth results from processes at work over millions of years and still at work today. Darwin's explanation for this great unfolding of life through time—the theory of evolution by natural selection—transformed our understanding of the living world, much as the ideas of Galileo, Newton, and Einstein revolutionized our understanding of the physical universe.

Darwin's theory of evolution by natural selection underlies all modern biology. It enables us to decipher our genes and fight viruses, and to understand Earth's fossil record and rich biodiversity. Simple yet at times controversial, misunderstood, and misused for social goals, the theory remains unchallenged as the central concept of biology. Charles Darwin, reluctant revolutionary, profoundly altered our view of the natural world and our place in it.

TheBarkerTheory.org

David Barker, MD, PhD, FRS is a physician and professor of clinical epidemiology at the University of Southampton, UK, and professor in the Department of Cardiovascular Medicine at the Oregon Health and Science University, US. Twenty years ago, he showed for the first time that people who had low birth weight are at greater risk of developing coronary heart disease. In 1995, the British Medical Journal named this the "Barker Hypothesis." It is now widely accepted. In 2010, *Time* magazine called it the "New Science." In 2003, he joined Professor Kent Thornburg at the faculty at the Heart Research Center, OHSU, to study how nutrition and growth before birth and during early childhood alter the development of the heart.

Dr. Barker's work is relevant to both Western countries and the developing world. In the Western world, many babies remain poorly nourished because their mothers eat diets that are unbalanced in macronutrients and deficient in micronutrients, or because their mothers are excessively thin or overweight. In the developing world, many girls and young women are chronically malnourished.

TheBarkerFoundation.org

The Barker Theory states that the way a baby grows in the womb affects its health in adult life.

In 1986, David Barker realized that areas of Britain currently recording high rates of coronary heart disease were the same areas that had recorded high rates of infant death seventy years before. The question he asked was: "Could it be that, in those areas with high infant mortality, the babies who clung to life had their development impaired in a way that made them vulnerable to heart disease as adults?"

The results of this study showed that there was a strong correlation between low birth weight and heart disease. An extensive search was undertaken to find old birth records, trace individuals, and establish their current health or cause of death. The results of this study showed that there was a strong correlation between low birth weight and heart disease. The work escalated, many papers were published, and studies were conducted worldwide adding to this body of knowledge. It became called the Barker Theory.

Low birth weight at full term indicates poor growth in the womb. Babies have low birth weight because they are undernourished. Other diseases have now been linked to low birth weight including diabetes, hypertension, stroke, osteoporosis and some cancers. The list continues to grow.

genographic.nationalgeographic.com

A Landmark Study of the Human Journey

Where do you really come from? And how did you get to where you live today? DNA studies suggest that all humans today descended from a group of African ancestors who—about sixty thousand years ago—began a remarkable journey.

amnh.org/exhibitions/permanent/other/evolution.html

American Museum of Natural History: Hall of Human Origins

The story of *Homo sapiens* is the topic of this hall, which explores human biology and anatomy, traces the path of human evolution, and examines the origins of human creativity. It is the only major exhibit in the country to present an in-depth investigation of the mysteries of human evolution.

The hall features four life-size dioramas of human predecessors *Australopithecus afarensis, Homo ergaster, Neanderthal,* and *Cro-Magnon,* showing each species in its habitat and demonstrating the behaviors and capabilities that scientists believe it had. Also displayed are full-sized casts of important fossils, such as the four-million-year-old "Lucy" skeleton and the 1.7-million-year-old "Turkana Boy," and *Homo erectus* specimens including a cast of "Peking Man." In addition, the hall features replicas of striking Ice Age art found in the Dordogne region of southwestern France. These beautiful limestone carvings of horses were made nearly twenty-six thousand years ago and represent what is believed to be the earliest artistic expression of humans.

mnh.si.edu

Smithsonian National Museum of Natural History

David H. Koch Hall of Human Origins

Based on decades of cutting-edge research by Smithsonian scientists, the David H. Koch Hall of Human Origins tells the epic story of human evolution and how humans evolved over six million years in response to a changing world. Following the process of scientific discovery, visitors will explore the evidence for human evolution, come face-to-face with unforgettable representations of early humans, and arrive at a deeper understanding of what it means to be human.

Bibliography

Abzhanov, Arhat, Winston P. Kuo, Christine Hartmann, et al. "The calmodulin pathway and evolution of elongated beak morphology in Darwin's finches." *Nature* 442-3 (August 2006).

Aiello L. C. and P. Wheeler. "The expensive-tissue hypothesis: the brain and the digestive system in human and primate evolution." *Current Anthropolgy* 46 (1995): 126-170.

Alberts, Bruce, Alexander Johnson, Julian Lewis, et al. *Molecular Biology of the Cell*. Garland Science, 2008.

Allis, C., David Jenuwein, Thomas Reinberg, et al., editors. *Epigenetics*. Cold Spring Harbor, New York: Cold Spring Harbor Laboratory Press, 2007.

Alvarez, H. P. "Grandmother Hypothesis and Primate Life Histories." *American Journal of Physical Anthropology* 113 (2000): 435-450.

American College of Sports Medicine, "Nutrition and Athletic Performance," position paper, 2000.

Anderson, Bob. *Stretching: For Everyday Fitness and for Running, Tennis, Racquetball, Cycling, Swimming, Golf, and Other Sports*. Bolinas, California: Shelter Publications, Inc., 1980.

Ard, Jamy D. "Unique Perspectives on the Obesogenic Environment." *Journal of General Internal Medicine* (July 2007).

Barker, David. *Nutrition in the Womb: How Better Nutrition During Development Will Prevent Heart Disease, Diabetes and Stroke.* The Developmental Origins of Health and Disease, 2008.

Barker, David. "The thrifty epigenotype: an acquired and heritable predisposition for obesity and diabetes." *Bioessays* 30(2) (2008): 156-66.

Barker, David, Johan G. Eriksson, Eero Kajantie, et al. "Boys Live Dangerously in the Womb." *American Journal of Human Biology* (October 2008).

Barton, Nicholas H., Derek E. G. Briggs, Jonathan Eisen, et al. *Evolution.* Cold Spring Harbor, New York: Cold Spring Harbor Laboratory Press, 2007.

Bass, Clarence. *Ripped: The Sensible Way to Achieve Ultimate Muscularity.* Ripped Enterprises, 1980.

Batmanghelidj, F. *Your Body's Many Cries for Water.* Global Health Solutions, 1997.

Beall, Cynthia M. "Andean, Tibetan, and Ethiopian patterns of adaptation to high-altitude hypoxia," from the symposium "Adaptations to Life at High Elevation" presented at the annual meeting of the Society for Integrative and Comparative Biology, January 4–8, 2005, at San Diego, California, Integrative and Comparative Biology, volume 46, number 1, pp. 18–24 January 6, 2006.

Biele, R., Y. Schutz, E. Jequier. "Energy metabolism during post exercise recovery in man." *The American Journal of Clinical Nutrition* 42 (July 1985): 69-82.

Bonner, John Tyler. *First Signals: The Evolution of Multicellular Development.* Princeton, New Jersey: Princeton University Press, 2000.

Bonner, John Tyler. *Why Size Matters: From Bacteria to . . . Blue Whales.* Princeton, New Jersey: Princeton University Press, 2006.

Brown, Janet. *Charles Darwin: Voyaging.* New Jersey: Princeton University Press, 1995.

Brown, Janet. *Charles Darwin: The Power of Place*. New Jersey: Princeton University Press, 2002.

Burke, Edmund R. *Optimal Muscle Performance and Recovery*. Avery, New York, 2003.

Callaway, Ewen. "Female Australopiths Left Home Once Mature, Males Didn't: Teeth from ancient human ancestors suggest that females joined new social groups once they reached maturity." *Nature* (2011).

Campbell, Neil A., and Jane B. Reece. *Biology*, Seventh Edition. San Francisco: Pearson, 2005.

Capellini, Isabella, Robert A. Barton, Patrick McNamara, et al. "Evolutionary importance of sleep: Phylogenetic analysis of the ecology and evolution of mammalian sleep." *Evolution* 62(7) (July 2008): 1764-1776.

Cline, John. "The Evolution of Sleep." *Psychology Today*, (March 2009).

Cohen, Gene D. *The Mature Mind: The Positive Power of the Aging Brain*. Basic Books, 2005.

Crespi, Erica, and Robert J. Denver. "Ancient Origins of Human Developmental Plasticity." *American Journal of Human Biology* 17 (2005): 44-54.

Csikszentmihalyi, Mihayli. *Flow: The Psychology of Optimal Experience*. Harper Perennial, 1990.

Darwin, Charles. *The Voyage of the Beagle: Charles Darwin's Journal of Research*. Pacific Publishing Studio, 1839.

Darwin, Charles. *The Origin of Species*. New York: Sterling, 1859.

Darwin, Charles, *The Descent of Man*, A Plume Book, 1871.

David, Yair Bar, Benjamin Gesundheit, Jacob Urkin, et al. "Water Intake and Cancer Prevention." *Journal of Clinical Oncology* 22(2) (January 15, 2004): 383-385.

Decker, H., K. E. Van Holde. *Oxygen and the Evolution of Life*. Berlin: Springer-Verlag, 2011.

DeGrasse Tyson, PhD, Neil. *Origins: Fourteen Billion Years of Cosmic Evolution*. NOVA, WBGH, Boston, 2004.

Desalle, Rob, and Ian Tattersall. *Human Origins: What Bones and Genomes Tell Us About Ourselves*. College Station, Texas: Texas A & M University Press, 2008.

Diamond, Jared. *The Third Chimpanzee: The Evolution and Future of the Human Animal*. Harper Perennial, 1992.

Di Pasquale, Mauro G. *Amino Acids and Proteins for the Athlete: The Anabolic Edge*. London: CRC Press, 2008.

Dudley, Robert. "Atmospheric oxygen, giant paleozoic insects and the evolution of aerial locomotor performance." *The Journal of Experimental Biology* 201 (1998): 1043-1050.

Edelson, Edward. *Gregor Mendel: And the Roots of Genetics*. Oxford University Press, 1999.

Erasmus, Udo. *Fats That Heal, Fats That Kill*. Alive Books, 1993.

Eriksson, J. G. "Early growth, and coronary heart disease and type 2 diabetes: experiences from the Helsinki Birth Cohort Studies." *International Journal of Obesity* 30 (2006): S18–S22.

Fagan, Brian M. *Human Prehistory and First Civilizations*. The Teaching Company, 2003.

Fernandez-Real, Jose Manuel, and Wifredo Ricart. "Insulin Resistance and Chronic Cardiovascular Inflammatory Syndrome." *Endocrine Reviews* 24(3) (2003): 278–301.

Finch, Caleb E. *The Biology of Human Longevity: Inflammation, Nutrition, and Aging in the Evolution of Lifespans*. Academic Press, 2007.

Flinna, Mark V., David C. Geary, and Carol V. Warda. "Ecological dominance, social competition, and coalitionary arms races: Why humans evolved extraordinary intelligence." *Evolution and Human Behavior* 26 (2005): 10-46.

Fogel, Robert William. *The Escape from Hunger and Premature Death,*

1700-2100: Europe, America, and the Third World. Cambridge University Press, 2004.

Food, Nutrition, Physical Activity, and the Prevention of Cancer: a Global Perspective, A Project of the World Cancer Research Fund International, 2007.

Fowler, Sharon P. "Even Diet Soda Induces Weight Gain in the Elderly." *Journal of Obesity* 16 (2008): 1894-1900.

Gibbons, Ann. *The First Human: The Race to Discover Our Earliest Ancestors.* New York: Anchor Books, 2006.

Goodsell, David S. *The Machinery of Life.* Springer, 2010.

Gluckman, Peter, and Mark Hanson. *The Fetal Matrix: Evolution, Development and Disease.* Cambridge University Press, 2005.

Gluckman, Peter D., Mark A. Hanson and Hamish G. Spencer. "Environmental influences during development and their later consequences for health and disease: implications for the interpretation of empirical studies." *Proceedings of the Royal Society* 272 (2005): 671-677.

Gluckman, Peter, and Mark Hanson. *Mismatch: The Lifestyle Diseases Timebomb.* Oxford University Press, 2008.

Gluckman, Peter, Alan Beedle, and Mark Hanson. *Principles of Evolutionary Medicine.* Oxford University Press, 2009.

Guarente, Leonard P., Linda Partridge, and Douglas C. Wallace. *The Molecular Biology of Aging.* Cold Spring Harbor, New York: Cold Spring Harbor Laboratory Press, 2008.

Haag, Marianne. "Essential Fatty Acids and the Brain." *Canadian Journal of Psychiatry* 48 (2003): 195–203.

Hager, Thomas. *Force of Nature: The Life of Linus Pauling.* New York: Simon & Schuster, 1995.

Halberstam, David. *The Amateurs: The Story of Four Young Men and Their Quest for an Olympic Gold Medal.* New York: Fawcell Books, 1985.

Hall, Sara. *Drawn to the Rhythm: A Passionate Life Reclaimed.* New York: W. W. Norton and Company, 2002.

Harris, Marvin, and Eric B. Ross. *Food and Evolution: Toward a Theory of Human Food Habits.* Philadelphia: Temple University Press, 1987.

Hawks, John. *The Rise of Humans: Great Scientific Debates.* The Teaching Company, 2011.

Hayflick, Leonard. *How and Why We Age.* New York: Ballantine Books, 1996.

Hazen, Robert M. *Origins of Life.* The Teaching Company, 2005.

Heymsfield, Steven B., Timothy G. Lohman, ZiMian Wang, et al., eds. *Human Body Composition.* Human Kinetics, 2005.

Heyward, Vivian H., and Lisa M. Stolarczyk. *Applied Body Composition Assessment.* Human Kinetics, 1996.

Higdon, Jane. *An Evidence-Based Approach to Vitamins and Minerals.* New York: Thieme, 2003.

Holt, Susanne, Janette C. Brand Miller, and Peter Petocz. "An insulin index of foods: the insulin demand generated by 1000-kJ portions of common foods." *American Journal of Clinical Nutrition* 66 (1997): 126.

Hu, Frank B. *Obesity Epidemiology.* Oxford University Press, 2008.

Hublin, Jean-Jacques, and Michael P. Richards, eds. *The Evolution of Hominin Diets: Integrating Approaches to the Study of Paleolithic Subsistence, a volume in the Max Planck Institute Subseries in Human Evolution.* Springer, 2009.

Hudson, Fredric M. *The Adult Years: Mastering the Art of Self-Renewal.* San Francisco: Jossey-Bass Publishers, 1991.

Huemer, Richard P., ed. *The Roots of Molecular Medicine: A Tribute to Linus Pauling.* New York: W. H. Freeman and Company, 1986.

Jablonka, Eva, and Marion J. Lamb. *Evolution in Four Dimensions: Genetic, Epigenetic, Behavioral, and Symbolic Variation in the History of Life.* Cambridge, Massachusetts: Massachusetts Institute of Technology, 2005.

Jobling, M. A., M. E. Hurles, and C. Tyler-Smith. *Human Evolutionary Genetics: Origins, Peoples & Disease*. Garland Science, 2004.

Johanson, Donald C., and Maitland Edey. *Lucy: The Beginnings of Humankind*. Simon & Schuster, 1981.

Johanson, Donald, and James Shreeve. *Lucy's Child: The Discovery of a Human Ancestor*. New York: William Morrow and Company, Inc., 1989.

Johanson, Donald, and Blake Edgar. *From Lucy to Language*. New York: Simon & Schuster, 2006.

Johanson, Donald C., and Kate Wong. *Lucy's Legacy: The Quest for Human Origins*. New York: Three Rivers Press, 2009.

Kandel, Eric R. *In Search of Memory: The Emergence of a New Science of Mind*. New York: W. W. Norton and Company, 2006.

Kaput, Jim, and Raymond L. Rodriguez, eds. *Nutritional Genomics: Discovering the Path to Personalized Nutrition*. Wiley-Interscience, 2006.

Kavanau, J. Lee. "Biological time-keeping mechanisms: A need for broader perspectives." *Medical Hypotheses* 67 (2006): 1258-1262.

Kavanau, J. Lee. "Is sleep's 'supreme mystery' unraveling? An evolutionary anaysis of sleep encounters no mystery; nor does life's earliest sleep, recently discovered in jellyfish." *Medical Hypotheses* 66 (2006): 3-9.

Kavanau, J. Lee. "Evolutionary approaches to understanding sleep." *Sleep Medicine Reviews* 9 (2005): 141-152.

Kavanau, J. Lee. "Evolutionary aspects of sleep and its REM and NREM states." *Advances in Cell Aging and Gerontology* 17 (2005): 1-32.

Kavanau, J. Lee. "Dream contents and failing memories." *Archives Italiennes de Biologie* 140 (2002): 109-127.

Kavanau, J. Lee. "REM and NREM sleep as natural accompaniments of the evolution of warm-bloodedness." *Neuriscience and Buibehavioral Reviews* 26 (2002): 889-906.

Kavanau, J. Lee. "Memory Failures, Dream Illusions and Mental Malfunction." *Neuropsychobiology* 26 (2001): 199-211.

Kavanau, J. Lee. "Adaptations and pathologies linked to dynamic stabilization of neural circuitry." *Neuroscience and Biobehavioral Reviews* 23 (1999): 635-648.

Kavanau, J. Lee. "Origin and evolution of sleep: Roles of vision and endothermy." *Brain Research Bulletin* 42 (1997): 245-263.

Kavanau, J. Lee. "Memory, sleep and the evolution of mechanisms of synaptic efficacy maintenance." *Neuroscience* 79.

Kiesling, Stephen, *The Shell Game: Reflections on Rowing and the Pursuit of Excellence*. Ashland, Oregon: Nordic Knight Press, 1982.

King, Barbara J. *Biological Anthropology: An Evolutionary Perspective*. The Teaching Company, 2002.

Klein, Richard G., and Blake Edgar. *The Dawn of Human Culture: A Bold New Theory of What Sparked the "Big Bang" of Human Consciousness*. John Wiley and Sons, Inc., 2002.

Klein, Richard G. *The Human Career: Human Biological and Cultural Origins*. Chicago: The University of Chicago Press, 2009.

Kolata, Gina. "Study Says Obesity Can Be Contagious." *New York Times*, July 25, 2007.

Lambert, Craig. *Mind Over Water: Lessons on Life from the Art of Rowing*. Boston: Houghton Mifflin Company, 1998.

Lake, Amelia A., Tim G. Townshend, and Seraphim Alvanides, eds. *Obesogenic Environments: Complexities, Perceptions, and Objective Measures*. Wiley-Blackwell, 2010.

Larbi, Anis, Claudio Franceschi, Dawn Mazzatti, et al. *Aging of the Immune System as a Prognostic Factor for Human Longevity*. Physiology 23 (2008):64-74.

Larson, Joan Matthews. *Seven Weeks to Sobriety: The Proven Program to Fight Alcoholism Through Nutrition*. Wellspring, New York: Ballantine, 1997.

Leakey, Richard, and Roger Lewin. *Origins Reconsidered: In Search of What Makes Us Human*. New York: Random House, 1992.

Levine, Benjamin D. "VO$_2$ Max: What do we know, and what do we still need to know?" *Journal of Physiology* 586.1 (2008): 25–34.

Levinson, Daniel J. *The Seasons of a Man's Life*. New York: Alfred A. Knopf, 1978.

Lindeberg, Staffan, S. Boyd Eaton, and Anthony Sebastian. "Origins and evolution of the Western diet: health implications for the 21st century." *American Journal of Clinical Nutrition* 81 (2005):341–54.

Lindeberg, Staffan. *Food and Western Disease: Health and Nutrition from an Evolutionary Perspective*. Wiley-Blackwell, 2010.

Liu, J., E. Head, A. Gharib, et al. "Delaying brain mitochondrial decay with mitochondrial antioxidants/metabolites, acetyl-L-carnitine and r-a-lipoic acid in old rats." *National Academy of Sciences*, 2002.

Lowry MD, and F. Stephen. "The Evolution of an Inflammatory Response." *Surgical Infections* 10(5) (October 2009): 419-425.

Maas, James B. *Power Sleep: The Revolutionary Program That Prepares Your Mind for Peak Performance*. Harper Collins, 1998.

Masoro, Edward J., and Steven N. Austad. *Handbook of the Biology of Aging*, Seventh Edition. Academic Press, 2011.

McArdle, William D., Frank I. Katch, and Victor L. Katch. *Essentials of Exercise Physiology*. Lippincott Williams & Wilkins, 2006.

McArdle, William D., Frank I. Katch, and Victor L. Katch. *Sports and Exercise Nutrition*. Lippincott Williams & Wilkins, 2009.

McKibben, Bill. *Long Distance: A Year of Living Strenuously*. New York: Simon & Schuster, 2000.

Mead, Clifford, and Thomas Hager. *Linus Pauling: Scientist and Peacemaker*. Oregon State Universtiy Press, 2001.

Medina, John. *Brain Rules: 12 Principles for Surviving and Thriving at*

Work, Home, and School. Pear Press, 2008.

Miller, Philip Lee. *The Life Extension Revolution: The New Science of Growing Older Without Aging.* Bantam Books, 2006.

Mintz, Sidney W. *Sweetness and Power: The Place of Sugar in Modern History.* Penguin Books, 1985.

Muehlenbein, Micahel. *Human Evolutionary Biology.* Cambridge University Press, 2010.

Neeson, Liam, narrator. *Evolution: Darwin's Dangerous Idea.* WGBH PBS, 2001.

Norden, Jeanette. *Understanding the Brain.* The Great Courses, 2007.

Northrup, Christiane. *The Wisdom of Menopause: Creating Physical and Emotional Health and Healing During the Change.* New York: Bantam Books, 2001.

Nova: *Cracking the Code of Life.* WGBH, Boston, 2004.

Nova: *Ghost in Your Genes.* WGBH, Boston, 2008.

Nova: *Becoming Human: How early hominids lived and evolved.* WGBH, Boston, 2009.

Nowicki, Stephen. *Biology: The Science of Life.* The Teaching Company, 2004.

Olson, Steve. *Mapping Human History: Discovering the Past Through Our Genes.* Bloomsbury, 2002.

Palmer, Douglas. Prehistoric *Past Revealed: The Four Billion Year History of Life on Earth.* Berkeley, California: University of California Press, 2003.

Palmer, Douglas. *Evolution: The Story of Life.* Berkeley, California: University of California Press, 2009.

Palmer, Douglas. *Origins: Human Evolution Revealed.* Mitchell Beazley, 2010.

Papas, Mia A., Anthony J. Alberg, Reid Ewing, et al. "The Built Environment and Obesity." *Epidemiologic Reviews* 29 (2007).

Pasiakos, S. M., H. L. McClung, J. P. McClung, et al. "Leucine-enriched essential amino acid supplementation during moderate steady state exercise enhances post exercise muscle protein synthesis." *American Journal of Clinical Nutrition* (2011).

Pauling, Linus. *How to Live Longer and Feel Better.* Avon Books, 1986.

Pauling, Linus. *Linus Pauling: In His Own Words.* Simon and Schuster, 1995.

Pigliucci, Massimo, and Jonathan Kaplan. *Making Sense of Evolution: The Conceptual Foundations of Evolutionary Biology.* Chicago: The University of Chicago Press, 2006.

Pigliucci, Massimo, and Gerd B. Muller, eds. *Evolution: The Extended Synthesis.* Cambridge, Massachusetts: MIT Press, 2010.

Potts, Richard, and Christopher Sloan. *What Does It Mean To Be Human?* National Geographic Society, 2010.

Power, Michael L., and Jay Schulkin. *The Evolution of Obesity.* Baltimore: The Johns Hopkins University Press, 2009.

Reaven, Gerald. *Syndrome X.* Simon and Schuster, 2001.

Rosenburg, Irwin, and William Evans. *Biomarkers: The 10 Determinants of Aging You Can Control.* Simon and Schuster, 1991.

Ruse, Michael. *Charles Darwin.* Blackwell Publishing, 2008.

Sanders, Robert. "Megavitamins may be useful treatment for many genetic diseases, or just good insurance to tune up body's metabolism." Report of Research of Bruce Ames, PhD, University of California, Berkeley, 2007.

Sapolsky, Robert M. *Why Zebras Don't Get Ulcers: An Updated Guide to Stress, Stress-Related Disease, and Coping.* New York: W. H. Freeman and Company, 1998.

Sapolsky, Robert M. *A Primate's Memoir: A Neuroscientist's Unconventional Life Among the Baboons*. New York: Scribner, 2001.

Schwartz, Leonard. *Heavyhands: The Ultimate Exercise*. Boston: Little, Brown and Company, 1982.

Schwartz, Leonard. *The Heavyhands Walking Book: An Open Invitation to Convert Walking into a Lifelong Total Fitness Strategy*. Panaerobics Press, 1990.

Sheehan, George. *Running & Being: The Total Experience*. Warner Books, 1978.

Silveira, Patricia P., Andre K. Portella, Marcelo Z. Goldani, et al. "Developmental origins of health and disease." *Journal of Pediatrics* (Nov./Dec. 2007).

Smith, John Maynard, and Eors Szathmary. *The Major Transitions in Evolution*. Oxford University Press, 1995.

Smith, John Maynard, and Eors Szathmary. *The Origins of Life: From the Birth of Life to the Origins of Language*. Oxford University Press, 1999.

Stanford, Craig B., and Henry T. Bunn, eds. *Meat-Eating and Human Evolution*. Oxford University Press, 2001.

Stanford, Craig B., John S. Allen, and Susan C. Anton. *Biological Anthropology*. New Jersey: Prentice Hall, 2006.

Stringer, Chris, and Peter Andrews. *The Complete World of Human Evolution*. London: Thames & Hudson, 2005.

Tan, Robert S. *Aging Men's Health: A Case-Based Approach*. New York: Thieme, 2005.

Tattersall, Ian. *Becoming Human: Evolution and Human Uniqueness*. New York: Harcourt Brace and Company, 1998.

Unger, Peter S., and Mark F. Teaford. *Human Diet: Its Origin and Evolution*. Westport, Connecticut: Bergin & Garvey, 2002.

Unger, Peter S., ed. *Evolution of the Human Diet: The Known, the Unknown, and the Unknowable*. Oxford University Press, 2007.

Wells, Jonathan C. K. *The Evolutionary Biology of Human Body Fatness: Thrift and Control.* Cambridge University Press, 2010.

Wells, Spencer. *The Journey of Man: A Genetic Odyssey.* New York: Random House, 2002.

Wells, Spencer. *Journey of Man: The Story of the Human Species.* PBS Home Video, 2003.

Wells, Spencer. *Deep Ancestry: Inside the Genographic Project.* National Geographic Society, 2006.

West, D. W., N. A. Burd, V. G. Coffey, et al. "Rapid aminoacidemia enhances myofibrillar protein synthesis and anabolic intramuscular signaling responses after resistance exercise." *American Journal of Clinical Nutrition* (2011).

West-Eberhard, Mary Jane. *Developmental Plasticity and Evolution.* Oxford University Press, 2003.

Willcox, D. Craig, J. Bradley, et al. "The Okinawan Diet: Health Implications of a Low-Calorie, Nutrient-Dense, Antioxidant-Rich Dietary Pattern Low in Glycemic Load." *Journal of the American College of Nutrition*, 28(4) (2009): 500S–516S.

Williams, David L., and Vincent Marks. *Scientific Foundations of Biochemistry in Clinical Practice* (Structure of pancreas & pancreatic system: 99% of the pancreas is devoted to handling the digestion of fats and protein while only 1% is devoted to handling sugar). Butterworth-Heinemann, 1994.

Wilmore, Jack H., and David L. Costill. *Physiology of Sport and Exercise.* Human Kinetics, 1999.

Wrangham, Richard. *Catching Fire: How Cooking Makes Us Human.* New York: Basic Books, 2009.

Wright, Robert. *The Moral Animal: Why We Are the Way We Are: The New Science of Evolutionary Psychology.* New York: Random House, 1994.

Wright, Robert. *Nonzero: The Logic of Human Destiny.* New York: Random House, 2000.

Wu, C. W., Y. C. Chen, and L. Yu. "Treadmill exercise counteracts the suppressive effects of peripheral lipopolysaccharide on hippocampal neurogenesis and learning and memory." *Journal of Neurochemistry.* December 103(6) (2007):2471-81.

Zimmer, Carl. *At the Water's Edge: Fish with Fingers, Whales with Legs, and How Life Came Ashore Then Went Back to Sea.* Simon & Schuster, 1998.

Zimmer, Carl. *Evolution: The Triumph of an Idea.* Harper Perennial, 2002.

Zimmer, Carl. *Soul Made Flesh: The Discovery of the Brain—and How it Changed the World.* New York: Free Press, 2004.

Zimmer, Carl. *Smithsonian Intimate Guide to Human Origins.* Smithsonian Books, 2005.

Zimmer, Carl. *The Tangled Bank: An Introduction to Evolution.* Greenwood Village, Colorado: Roberts and Company, 2010.

Index